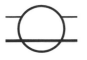

# DISABILITY DISCOURSE

**Disability, Human Rights and Society**
Series Editor: Professor Len Barton, University of Sheffield

The *Disability, Human Rights and Society* series reflects a commitment to a particular view of 'disability' and a desire to make this view accessible to a wider audience. The series approach defines a 'disability' as a form of oppression and identifies the ways in which disabled people are marginalized, restricted and experience discrimination. The fundamental issue is not one of an individual's inabilities or limitations, but rather a hostile and unadaptive society.

Authors in this series are united in the belief that the question of disability must be set within an equal opportunities framework. The series gives priority to the examination and critique of those factors that are unacceptable, offensive and in need of change. It also recognizes that any attempt to redirect resources in order to provide opportunities for discriminated people cannot pretend to be apolitical. Finally, it raises the urgent task of establishing links with other marginalized groups in an attempt to engage in a common struggle. The issue of disability needs to be given equal significance to those of race, gender and age in equal opportunities policies. This series provides support for such a task.

Anyone interested in contributing to the series is invited to approach the Series Editor at the Division of Education, University of Sheffield.

*Current and forthcoming titles*

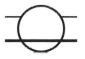

# DISABILITY DISCOURSE

Edited by
**Mairian Corker and Sally French**

**Open University Press**
Buckingham · Philadelphia

Open University Press
Celtic Court
22 Ballmoor
Buckingham
MK18 1XW

email: enquiries@openup.co.uk
world wide web: http://www.openup.co.uk

and
325 Chestnut Street
Philadelphia, PA 19106, USA

First Published 1999

A catalogue record of this book is available from the British Library

ISBN    0 335 20222 5 (pb)    0 335 20223 3 (hb)

*Library of Congress Cataloging-in-Publication Data*
Disability discourse / Mairian Corker and Sally French (eds).
        p.    cm.    — (Disability, human rights and society)
     Includes bibliographical references and index.
     ISBN 0-335-20223-3 (hbk). — ISBN 0-335-20222-5 (pbk)
     1. Disability studies.    2. Sociology of disability.    3. Handicapped.    I. Corker,
        Mairian.    II. French, Sally. III.    Series
     HV1568.2.D57    1999
     305.9'08—dc21                                                98-20844
                                                                           CIP

Copy-edited and typeset by The Running Head Limited, London and Cambridge
Printed in Great Britain by St Edmundsbury Press, Bury St Edmunds

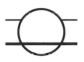

# Contents

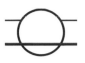

# Notes on contributors

**Simone Aspis** is a former assistant with the BBC Radio 4 Programme *Does He Take Sugar?* and Parliamentary and Campaigns Officer for People First, where she rewrote the parliamentary Civil Rights (Disabled Persons) Bill in pictorial and simple text format so that disabled people with the learning difficulties label could have access to its contents. She now runs her own consultancy, Changing Perspectives.

**Dona Avery** is completing her doctorate in English at Arizona State University. She is currently a Visiting Scholar at Bristol University, evaluating disability studies programmes in the UK. Her experience of disability is informed by personal familiarity with cerebral palsy and multiple sclerosis, as well as by academic conclusions that situate disability issues as being parallel to the oppression encountered by ethnic minorities and women.

**Sue Boazman** has taken part in a number of major innovative projects for people with aphasia since she experienced a stroke in 1989, including the Joseph Rowntree Foundation-funded project, 'Talking About Aphasia', conducted by staff at the Department of Clinical Communication Studies at the City University, London. She is one of only three aphasic counsellors in the UK.

**Brenda Jo Brueggemann** is an assistant professor (of English and Comparative Studies) at The Ohio State University, where she teaches courses in rhetoric, non-fiction writing, literacy studies and disability studies. She has published numerous essays in the US on disability and deafness and is author of the forthcoming *Lend Me Your Ear: Rhetorical Constructions of Deafness*. She is currently working on a new project, 'Women, Authority, Deafness: Constructing Literate Lives', which examines the nature and development of (female) authority in deaf women professionals. Brenda Jo is hard-of-hearing from birth.

**Brad Byrom** is a PhD candidate in the Department of History at the University of Iowa, USA. He has spent much of the last eight years conducting research into the history of disability, and is currently completing a dissertation on the topic of 'Physical Disability in the United States between 1900 and 1940'.

**Colin Cameron** works in North Tyneside as manager of Tyneside Disability Arts. He has recently been involved in writing a disability studies degree course for the University of Northumbria at Newcastle, and is researching a PhD on the cultural history of the disability arts movement.

**Mairian Corker** is currently a part-time Senior Research Fellow at the University of Central Lancashire and Research Associate on the ESRC-funded project, 'Life as a Disabled Child', coordinated by the Universities of Edinburgh and Leeds. Deaf herself, she is author of numerous books, articles and distance learning materials on deaf and disability studies, including *Deaf Transitions* and *Deaf and Disabled, or Deafness Disabled?*, and is editor of *Deaf Worlds* and an executive editor of *Disability and Society*.

**James A. Fredal** is an assistant professor of English at The Ohio State University. He teaches courses in rhetoric, writing and biblical literature, and has recently completed a dissertation on classical rhetoric, 'Beyond the Fifth Canon: The Construction of Speech in Classical Rhetoric'. There he investigates the way in which speech is 'normalized' throughout the development of rhetoric (and thus, in our culture) and interrogates the way a disabled body performs speech and delivers rhetoric.

**Sally French** works as a lecturer at Brunel University and as a freelance writer, lecturer and physiotherapist. She has written and edited many articles and books on disability issues, including *On Equal Terms* (published by Butterworth-Heinemann), and was involved in writing and developing the Open University Course *Disabling Society – Enabling Interventions*.

**Susan Gabel** is an Assistant Professor of Education at The University of Michigan-Flint, where she teaches courses in educational foundations and disability studies. Her doctorate is from Michigan State University, in curriculum, teaching and educational policy. Her current research is in critical disability theory with a postmodernist perspective. Her most recent projects include a forthcoming book, *Pedagogy and an Aesthetic of Disability*, and a set of case studies examining the connections between personal and professional identities of people undergoing significant identity transformations.

**Anthony Hogan** is a postdoctoral Research Fellow in the faculty of Health Sciences, University of Sydney. He has worked as an activist, sociologist and rehabilitation counsellor with Deaf and Deafened people in Australia for the last 12 years. He has been involved in the development of a variety of services and policy documents addressing the concerns of these communities.

**Mike Oliver** is Professor of Disability Studies at the University of Greenwich, UK. He is an internationally recognized academic and political commentator, having participated in several major policy reviews in education, health and social services and published numerous books and articles on disability and other social policy issues over the last 20 years. He has also made many appearances on national and regional television and radio. He is also a political activist and a member of the disability movement. His most recent books are on the history and significance of the disability movement and social policy and disability.

**Susan Peters** received her PhD from Stanford University in 1987 with emphasis on educational administration and policy analysis. Prior to this, she taught in primary schools in Tokyo, Japan and Los Angeles, California. She is a disability rights activist, having held leadership positions in the Independent Living Movement in the US, and participated in the disability rights movement in Zimbabwe. She is a former Fulbright scholar whose interests include African studies, disability studies, and comparative studies in education. She is currently an Associate Professor at the College of Education, Michigan State University, US.

**Mark Priestley** is a Research Fellow in the Disability Research Unit at the University of Leeds and administrator of the international discussion group disability-research@mailbase.ac.uk. He was formerly a lecturer in rehabilitation work with visually impaired people and an independent trainer with social services staff.

**Tom Shakespeare** is a Research Fellow at the Disability Research Unit, University of Leeds. A member of the disability movement, he has written widely on aspects of disabled identity, culture and politics, and, more recently, on genetics. He is co-author of *The Sexual Politics of Disability* and editor of *The Disability Reader*.

**Murray Simpson** is a lecturer at the University of Dundee, Department of Social Work. His particular research interests include the history and sociology of the discourse of learning disability. He is currently researching the treatment of 'idiocy' in the nineteenth century for his doctorate.

**Judy Singer** is currently writing an honours thesis at the University of Technology, Sydney. Her research interests include the varying accounts of children of disabled parents/parents of disabled children/disabled adults, autism as a metaphor, autism and the language of cybernetics, and autistic uses of the Internet. Both her mother and her daughter have autism.

**Sandy Slack** is a former physical education teacher in secondary education and has worked extensively in the voluntary sector both locally and nationally. She has been a National Association of Volunteer Bureaux committee member and volunteer for 13 years and is now a freelance consultant trainer in disability equality and staff development. She is an Associate Lecturer at the Open University's School of Health and Social Welfare.

**Emma Stone** was until recently based at the Disability Research Unit, University of Leeds. She is nearing completion of her PhD thesis on disability and development in China. She has recently undertaken consultancy work with Save the Children Fund UK and UNICEF-China, organized the first UK Forum on Disability and Development in the Majority World, and been the principal researcher on the Disability Research Unit's Snowdon Survey project, which aims to identify financial and information barriers to disabled people's participation in post-16 study.

**John Swain** is a Senior Lecturer in the Faculty of Health, Social Work and Education, University of Northumbria, UK. He contributed to the production of the Open University Course *The Handicapped Person in the Community* as a course team member. He has written extensively, particularly on issues concerning learning disability and visual impairment.

**Carol Thomas** is a lecturer in the Department of Applied Social Science at Lancaster University, and is centrally involved in the University's Institute for Health Research. She is a sociologist who has researched, published and taught in disability studies in recent years. She currently has a Leverhulme Trust Research Fellowship to enable her to complete her forthcoming book (to be published in this series) on disability theory and disabled women's experiences.

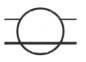

# Series editor's preface

The Disability, Human Rights and Society series reflects a commitment to a social model of disability and a desire to make this view accessible to a wide audience. 'Disability' is viewed as a form of oppression and the fundamental issue is not one of an individual's inabilities or limitations, but rather, a hostile and unadaptive society.

Priority is given to identifying and challenging those barriers to change, including the urgent task of establishing links with other marginalized groups and thus seeking to make connections between class, gender, race, age and disability factors.

The series aims to further establish disability as a serious topic of study, one in which the latest research findings and ideas can be seriously engaged with.

This edited collection represents the sheer range of ideas now being discussed within disability studies. It is also an attempt to contribute to the development of alternative conceptions, including interpretations of (for example) the relationship between disability and impairment.

The different stages of development and commitment to the key ideas being advocated is reflected in the levels of analysis and interpretation that the different contributors offer. However, all of them have a concern to raise questions that have personal, political and professional significance in their lives.

The papers both raise questions about single-issue identity politics and emphasize the establishment of a disability discourse that is multi-layered and able to reflect voices which, it is claimed, have been hitherto silenced, borderline or unfamiliar.

By encouraging a cross-fertilization of ideas and by being sensitive to the importance of historical, cultural difference and context, the book advocates a form of discourse that will, it is hoped, generate new knowledge and support and pursue innovatory ways of exploring the experience of disability.

The book is a thoughtful and challenging read, one which I have no doubt will stimulate debate and critical responses. The issues are complex and contentious; the editors hope that the book will contribute to the generation of creative and imaginative engagement, and will be a resource which can be actively drawn upon as part of the fundamental struggle to challenge oppression and discrimination in the lives of disabled people.

I too share this hope.

Professor Len Barton
Sheffield

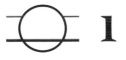 **1**

# Reclaiming discourse in disability studies

## Mairian Corker and Sally French

> Practising cultural studies involves constantly redefining it in response to changing geographical and historical conditions, and to changing political demands. [It] always has to begin again by turning to discourses as both its productive entrance into and productive dimension of that context. In the end, it is not interested in the discourse per se but in the articulations between everyday life and the formations of power. Discourses are ... active agents, not even merely performances, in the material world of power.
>
> (Grossberg 1998: 67–8, 75)

### Introduction

This book resulted from a chance meeting between us some years ago. It was the first opportunity that we had had to engage in in-depth discussions about each other both personally, politically and professionally. On one level, it was clear from the outset that language was a critical, even conflictual issue for both of us on account of our different professional backgrounds and disciplines. We used different languages in our work and in our writing and were often writing for different audiences and about different issues. Further we communicated with each other from different and often contested positions in the communicative web. One of us needed dim lighting and the other bright and even lighting, one of us was visual whereas the other was aural; one of us was dependent on the nuances of body language while the other was unable to detect these nuances and reflect them in her communication. We became aware, through reading each other's writing, that, on another level, our worlds were also made up of overarching and totalizing discursive practices which objectified and defined one of us as 'hearing impaired' and the other as 'visually impaired', while systematically disabling us by silencing what was undoubtedly a *shared meaning* and the way in which we had individually and socially authored our own lives. We found this shared meaning in our collective experience of disability oppression. But there remained some niggling questions around whether disability theory was inclusive of the particular ways in which we conceptualized our shared meaning of disability oppression.

## Dilemmas of disability theory

Social model theory rests on the distinction between disability, which is socially created, and impairment, which is referred to as a physical attribute of the body. In this sense it establishes a paradigm for disabled people which is equivalent to those of sex/gender and race/ethnicity. However, though it is a ground-breaking concept, and one which has provided tremendous political impetus for disabled people, we feel that because the distinction between disability and impairment is presented as a dualism or dichotomy – one part of which (disability) tends to be valorized and the other part (impairment) marginalized or silenced – social model theory, itself, produces and embodies distinctions of value and power. For example, Paul Anthony Darke (1998a: 224) in a recent book review says: 'There is no such group as people with disabilities; there are people with impairments and disabled people, but they are quite distinct things: linguistically, politically and theoretically.'

We do not dispute this as being an accurate description of the social model theory. However, it does contain a contradiction in terms which risks weakening the model's theoretical power. In saying that 'people with impairments' and 'disabled people' are 'quite distinct things', the conceptual link between impairment and *disability oppression* is broken because it could be construed that disability and impairment *are not related*. To paraphrase Ingraham (1996: 183), this 'reinforces the nature/culture binary', opening the study of impairment to the domain of science and closing off consideration of how 'biology is linked to culture'. Impairment as a biological category escapes the realm of construction or achieved status, even though it is, itself, 'defined' or 'constructed'. If disability is indeed a form of social oppression, the questions then remain – 'Oppression *of what or whom?*' and '*Why and how does this particular form of oppression occur?*' It is our view that we cannot adequately answer these questions without addressing impairment.

The reason why this is important for the current volume is that these dichotomies come to be reflected in discourses – 'as linguistic systems of statements through which we speak of ourselves and our social world' (Leonard 1997: 2). Thus the 'disabled body' is a site of discursive production *and* consumption:

> The articulation of discourses about 'problems' takes the form of a political arena in which sets of activities, discursive and material, have mutual effects. So, a discourse on a problem within the field of welfare (for example 'dependency on state financial benefits') is not constituted

simply as a system of statements or a set of questions, a discourse about the 'real world', but is immediately caught up in a set of material practices (the activities of social security claimants and officials, for example) which are a historical project . . . Discourses, in other words, are constructed through linguistic rules and social practices which direct our attention to the politics of knowledge-producing activities.

(Leonard 1997: 11–12)

Thus the material world of economics and the socio-cultural world as mediated by discourse are intricately enmeshed (Laclau and Mouffe 1990), but this idea does not rest easily within theories and practice which concentrate on one or the other. Nevertheless, the importance of discourse as a knowledge-producing activity becomes clear when we note that impairment is removed from the equation in three overlapping ways, all of which make use of discursive strategies:

- By 'the language and politics of exclusion' (Riggins 1997) or omission, which in linguistics is referred to as *elision*. Here, whereas 'impairment' is only an attribute or identity, disability is a framework of differential analysis and a primary way of signifying relationships of power. Thus impairment becomes a fixed surface onto which disability is projected by 'culture'.
- Because impairment is also a referent for the 'individual', 'medical' and 'administrative' models of disability, this commonality must be denied. This strategy is implicit in the suggestion that we must not talk about impairment because this 'allows those who wish to see disability as personal, pathological and impairment-specific an opportunity to use a misappropriation of the social model of disability as justification for preventing or blocking disability equality' (Darke 1998a: 224).
- This is achieved through the production of a division of meaning (semantic splitting) of 'impairment' and the redistribution of its constituent parts in such a way that the boundaries between disability and impairment are blurred. For example, *disability* is more accurately described by terms such as wheelchair user, Braille reader and hearing aid user, and impairment by terms such as mobility impaired, visually impaired and hearing impaired. However, the latter terms are frequently used as descriptors for the former, thus conflating disability and impairment.

Oliver (1996b: 44) is quite right when he says that the struggles around language are not merely 'semantic'. The problem with strategies which effectively ask us to choose between the extremes of 'reality determinism' and 'discourse determinism' (Leonard 1997: 11) is that they produce a situation where disability appears to be, as Lane (1995: 179) suggests, 'lying there in the road', created out of nothing, while impairment 'belongs' in medical textbooks (Lane *et al.* 1997) and individualized politics which reinforce the dominant discourse of disability. This discourse also conflates disability and impairment to produce further semantic problems:

for the social model of disability, the body – reduced to impairment – finds itself, inescapably, in the jurisdiction of medicine. The relationship of disabled people to their bodies is mediated by medicine and therapy, and has nothing to do with policy and politics. This dualistic approach produces a theoretical rigidity which involves the medicalisation of disabled peoples' bodies and the politicisation of their social lives. There is a theoretical closure around the relationship between sociology and the body which makes a sociology of impairment unthinkable.

(Hughes and Paterson 1997: 331)

This presupposition is one reason why, though we agree that social model theory is not intended to embrace impairment, we feel that Oliver's (1996b) notion of a separate sociology of impairment will not work. Because social model theory is framed in the way that it is, it will work directly against a sociology of impairment, inhibiting its development in exactly the same way that the dominant framework of feminism (which separates sex from gender and places *gender* at its centre) thwarts the work of a gay and lesbian studies (which has *sex* at its centre and distinguishes it from sexuality) (Butler 1997).

Since disability and impairment are clearly discursively related (that is, in practice it is very difficult to 'talk' about disability without referring to impairment, and because 'the impaired body' is both a site of discourse production and a site onto which cultural discourses are projected), such practice marginalizes the role of discourse in creating *and challenging* disability oppression. When framed in this terminology, the 'social body' is reduced to a material dimension – to 'physical capital' (Bourdieu 1986) which is then translated into (materialist) economic, cultural or social capital, for example. Discourses of 'the body' are in themselves something of an anathema to us. Certainly, talking about 'the body' is relevant to us as disabled *women*, but social model theory employs the same strategies given above to marginalize feminist views of disability, and so this particular configuration of 'body talk' is rendered meaningless. But more importantly, the presupposition that the boundary between disability and impairment is solid does not allow us to explore adequately our experience of disability oppression because this experience is 'in between' – discursively produced at the interface of society and the individual – and neither of us feels that the barriers we experience as disabled people can be regarded as either 'entirely socially produced or amenable to social action' (French 1993: 17). At best, we have 'leaky bodies and boundaries' (Shildrick 1997), and as a result there is a tendency for social model theory to problematize, and therefore dismiss, our disabilities 'without solutions' as 'impairments' (French 1993: 23).

If, as Oliver (1990, 1996a) and others suggest, disability is *only* a consequence of material relations between the body and culture, then it is unsurprising that 'solutions' to disability oppression cited in the application of social model theory *are* often impairment-specific (Corker 1998), and frequently technological (in the case of people with visual and hearing impairments, minicoms, beeper crossings and so on). So there is a sense in which we see the *exclusive* employment of the material as an attempt to dehumanize us. This view is not unreasonable or theoretically unsound. It is another dimension to disability theory, for, as some of the contributions in this book show, the dominant discourse on disability attributes negative ascriptions to people who have too close a relationship with technology, in part as a result of valorization of the notion of autonomy from others in Western society (Latour 1992; Lakoff 1995; Lupton 1995; Turkle 1996; Lupton and Noble 1997). This is reminiscent of Deveaux's (1994: 227) view that cultural practices have the effect of 'diminishing and delimiting women's subjectivity, at times treating women as robotic receptacles of culture rather than as active agents who are both constituted by, and reflective of their social and cultural contexts'. Technological solutions to disability can therefore be *a significant factor in our oppression*. Further, the social model framework reduces phenomenological notions of the embodied Self – that is, notions which see the relationship between mind and body as symbiotic and relational (see, for example, Shakespeare 1994) – and discourses of mind (Shilling 1993; Bendelow and Williams 1995), emotion (Parkinson 1995; Harré and Parrott 1996) and sensation (Shilling and Mellor 1996; Corker 1998) to the margins alongside, perhaps even embodied in 'biological impairment'.

This is particularly problematic for many disabled people because 'the impaired body' is not always fully visible; nor indeed is impairment always 'bodily' in the material sense, as some of the contributors to this book highlight. For example, we would argue that there is a huge difference between a Deaf person who uses sign language and/or has 'deaf speech' and a deaf person who uses a hearing aid and communicates well orally; but this difference cannot always be concretely described in terms of disability or impairment. It is moreover interesting to observe how the term 'disabled' is applied (or not) in these two cases (Corker 1998). It is also problematic for our analysis of particular aspects of disability and impairment. For example, Barnes on the one hand says that phenomenological accounts of disability reduce 'explanations for cultural phenomena such as perceptions of physical, sensory and intellectual difference to the level of thought processes' (1996: 49), which is a reductionist reading of phenomenology focused on the work of phenomenologists such as Merleau Ponty (1962) who sought to stand realism on its head. On the other, he asserts that:

> this essentially individualistic approach might be an appropriate remedy for those sections of the disabled community *who do experience physical pain as a consequence of their impairment, but what of those who don't? Examples include blind people, deaf people, people with epilepsy, people of short stature or people with learning difficulties* . . . I have little doubt that [Wendell, *The Rejected Body*] will be welcomed by the true confessions brigade; those intent on writing about themselves rather than engaging in serious political analysis of a society that is inherently disabling.
>
> (Barnes 1998: 146)

Any deaf person who lives with tinnitus – 'noises in the head' which can be so severe and controlling that they cause mental illness, or recruitment: a 'physical' phenomenon which makes loud sounds painful and sometimes renders the 'material' solution of hearing aids ineffective – would dispute that deaf people don't experience physical pain as a consequence of their impairments. Further, some conditions which result in blindness can also be physically painful – for example, the pressure created in the eyes by glaucoma – and many visually and hearing-impaired people are prone to intermittent headaches. It is not easy in situations such as this to locate pain within impairment or disability.

Research shows, however, that pain is never the sole creation of our anatomy and physiology (French 1997). Rather, as Morris (1991: 1) suggests, it emerges only at 'the intersection of bodies, minds and cultures'. Barnes therefore demolishes his earlier argument with discursive generalizations – that is totalizing terms which disguise real differences – in suggesting that certain *groups* of disabled people don't feel pain *per se*, in part because pain is assumed to be 'physical', chronic and, most importantly, lacking a 'cultural' dimension. By extension, if these multiple influences are ignored, then what is being referred to is impairment and not disability. Secondly, Barnes's reference to 'the true confessions brigade' suggests that only collective analysis is 'serious political analysis'. The assumption that 'personal' narratives can only be 'read' at a personal level seems to challenge one of the fundamental tenets of new social movements – namely, that the personal is, may be or must be the political (Morris 1991; Oliver 1996a; Shilling 1997).

## Reclaiming discourse

To summarize so far then, much of the uneasiness that we have with the current framework of disability theory stems from its failure to conceptualize a mutually constitutive relationship between impairment and disability which is both materially and discursively (socially) produced. When used in this way, social model theory cannot 'address the political crisis of ecology in significant and compelling ways' (Grossberg 1998: 70) because it takes a narrow view of the power of discursive practices. Though it recognizes the close links between 'knowledge about language and discourse, and power', it has not yet been 'refined on the basis of the anticipated effects of . . . the finest details of linguistic choices [which] bring about discursive change through conscious design' (Fairclough 1993: 216). There have, of course, been many attempts to challenge the dominance of these ways of thinking, philosophically (Derrida 1978; Halliday 1978; Foucault 1979; Pêcheux 1982, 1988; Ricœur 1992), and specifically within medical sociology/health studies (Lupton 1994; Radley 1994; Tudor 1996; Bury 1997; Yardley 1997) and disability studies (Barnes and Mercer 1996; Bury 1996; Oliver 1996a; Johnston 1997; Pinder 1997; Mitchell and Snyder 1997; Shakespeare and Watson 1997; Corker 1998). But such attempts are preoccupied with questions of *who* should do research and whether research is 'objective' or 'subjective', the *right* way to study disability, and how to define 'discourse', 'the body', and 'culture' for example; many reproduce the reductionisms and boundary-marking which threaten both their theoretical integrity and their political effectiveness. Many of these questions themselves have a discursive dimension.

Hence we find ourselves caught in the middle of a modern paradox – a 'crisis of representation' (Hennessy 1993). But why do we now find ourselves looking to Western culture's 'linguistic turn' in social theory for solutions? And what, indeed, does impairment have to do with disability?

To counter the kind of discourses described in the previous two sections is critical for us, personally and politically, as people with sensory impairments and as disabled women. It is also, we feel, important intellectually to the discipline of disability studies, as the debates surrounding these issues form a considerable part of the analytical basis of contemporary mainstream social theory, and we do not want disability to be excluded from mainstream analysis. It is at this point, then, that we must make a distinction between disability studies and social model theory. Disability studies, as we understand it, certainly includes and is founded on social model theory, but it is clear that social model theory does not embrace contemporary disability studies in its entirety, nor does it include all disabled people (Oliver 1996a). One of the arguments put forward in Oliver's book is that the conflation of the two results from a failure on the part of some disability theorists to engage in the reflexive redefinition of disability (in the social model sense) according to changing knowledges, contexts and cultures. For example, it is not true to say that Oliver's 'conception of material relations is *fully* inclusive of socio-cultural factors' (Darke 1998: 223, italics added) in the context of changing knowledges about and understandings of 'culture' (Corker 1998; 1999, forthcoming).

Returning to the 'modern paradox', then, our answer to the first question is that, for disability studies, this paradox is contained in questions about the *reciprocal relationships* between the discursive, and therefore socio-cultural aspects of our experience as disabled people and our material existence in a disabling society. For example, we might endeavour to discover how the practical consequences of hearing impairment, such as the inability to understand voice announcements at a railway station, affect the identity and social relationships of hearing-impaired people? Conversely, how do beliefs about the material aspects of hearing impairment (that hearing aids eliminate hearing impairment, or that someone who does not sign must be hearing) influence the activities and opportunities of hearing-impaired people? This assumes that disability is discursively and materially created – hence the answer to the second question.

This is addressed succinctly in the work of Norman Fairclough (1993, 1995). He stresses the importance of discourse analysis as a method for studying social change. But he notes (1993: 1) that the necessary synthesis of linguistic analysis and 'social and political thought relevant to developing an adequate social theory of language' required for this has faced many barriers.

For example, linguistics, itself 'dominated by formalistic and cognitive paradigms', has been isolated from other social sciences which tend to see language as 'transparent'. But the boundaries between social sciences have been weakening, which has resulted in language being accorded a more central role in social phenomena. Fairclough stresses, moreover, that it is important to hang on to the role of language in ideology (Althusser 1971; Gramsci 1971), representation and social reproduction, and so language must be viewed as a powerful mechanism for social and cultural change.

> We are witnessing a 'technologization of discourse' (Fairclough 1990) in which discursive technologies as a type of 'technologies of government' (Rose and Miller 1989) are being systematically applied in a variety of organizations by professional technologists who research, redesign and provide training in discourse practices.
>
> (Fairclough 1993: 8)

Fairclough is primarily referring here to modern discourse technologies such as interviewing, teaching, counselling and advertising, which are employed by 'powerholders' in the services of social control because they are seen as 'transcontextual' resources and toolkits designed to have particular effects upon 'publics (clients, customers and consumers) who are not trained in them' (1993: 215–16). For example, one of us has argued that there is a very fine dividing line between counselling which promotes social-emotional re-education, and counselling which promotes 'normalcy' in relation to deaf people, because the dominant discourse of some approaches to counselling can view a fully self-actualized person as someone who behaves in a 'socially acceptable' or 'normal' way and promotes this as the 'solution' to the client's problem (Corker 1994). The same could be said of 'special needs' teaching practice which promotes 'normalization' rather than education. Habermas (1984: xi) has described this in terms of the colonization of the 'lifeworld' by the 'systems' of the state and the economy.

However, as Henriques *et al.* (1984: 106) point out, 'discourses delimit what can be said, whilst providing the spaces – the concepts, metaphors, models, analogies – for making new statements'. In other words, every discursive technology has within it implicit counter-technologies which can compete with it in the public domain. Counter-technologists include those who have re-authored theories of gender (Crawford 1995; Cheshire and Trudgill 1998; Coates 1998), race (van Dijk 1987; Wetherell and Potter 1992), sexuality (Plummer 1995; Seidman 1996) in ways which *resist* hegemonic discourses. Indeed, in the field of disability studies, the social model is a classic example of re-authoring. However, to make this 'critical' function of discourse more visible it is necessary to reclaim it – to place it, perhaps temporarily, at the centre of disability theory and to analyse what happens when we do this in a variety of different ways. We are aware of the risks associated with such an exercise as, in returning us to the question of impairment, they have been well articulated in explorations of the category 'woman' and its relationship to feminism:

woman is a simultaneous foundation of and irritant to feminism . . . It is true that the trade-off for the myriad namings of 'women' by politics, sociologies, policies and psychologies is that at this cost women do some-times become a force to be reckoned with. But the caveat remains: The risky elements to the processes of alignment in sexed ranks are never far away, and the very collectivity which distinguishes you may also be wielded, even unintentionally, against you. Not just against you as an individual, that is, but against you as a social being with needs and attri-butions. The dangerous intimacy between subjectivity and subjectifica-tion needs careful calibration.

(Riley 1988: 17)

However, we do not believe that this is a threat to social model theory, because fundamental to the achievement of 'careful calibration' of this exer-cise is a view of 'text' – a term which refers to anything which can be 'read', including material artifacts – as being multi-layered and multi-dimensional, a view which, we believe, is supported by the multiple and often conflicting interpretations which are given to most 'texts', even within disability studies. This embraces Fairclough's notion that:

Any discursive 'event' . . . is seen as being simultaneously a piece of text, an instance of discursive practice, and an instance of social practice . . . The 'social practice' dimension attends to issues of concern in social analysis such as the institutional and organizational circumstances of the discursive events and how that shapes the nature of the discursive practice, and the constitutive/constructive effects of discourse.

(Fairclough 1993: 4)

This is an important concept, which has been emphasized by writers in other fields (for example, Langellier 1989; Finnegan 1992; McLeod 1997), and which highlights some of the deficiencies in existing approaches to the study of disability discourse. Within disability theory, there have been two main strands of analysis which influence the way in which the relationship between the personal and the political is seen. First, there is often a tendency to regard the authoring and audiencing of 'texts' as unchanging and static, so that they are seen as 'finished products [with] little attention to processes of text production and interpretation, or the tensions which characterise these processes'. Such an approach makes it difficult to 'investigate language *dynamically* within processes of social and cultural change' (Fairclough 1993: 2, italics added). This criticism applies to Barnes's earlier comments. Second, discursive analysis of disability focuses either on 'surface' semantics – the 'superficial' and 'observable' level of expression (van Dijk 1997: 6) – and 'playful' postmodernism (Corbett 1996: 101) which risks creating chaotic fragmentation, or on ideology and hegemony (Oliver 1996a). This means that the analysis of disability discourse lacks a 'reflexive' component which emphasizes that 'it is not always possible, or desirable, to neatly distinguish between doing "value-free" and technical discourse analysis on the one hand, and engaging in social, cultural or political critique on the other' (van Dijk 1997: 23).

Applying this to our own contexts (and by way of response to Barnes's criticisms), we feel, both as disabled people who have written *in* the personal (French 1993, 1994) and as disabled people who have, at times, given the personal narratives prominence in our writing (Corker 1994, 1996), that we, like Barnes, are attempting to 'uncover, demystify or otherwise challenge [the] dominance' (van Dijk 1997: 22) of ways of conflating disability and impairment which insist that both the 'problem' and the 'solution' are always our individual responsibility.

However, we do this from a different position, and we wish to make that clear. When we write in this way, or encourage others to tell their stories, we are emphatically *not* inviting our oppressors to say 'We told you so!' for *we are not always writing with them in mind*; nor do we see disabled people's stories as solely props for the 'true confessions brigade'. How these stories are interpreted surely depends on who the audience is and, as Davis (1995: xi) notes, 'books about disability are usually little read; academic sessions at professional conferences, and other types of meeting about disability are usually poorly attended'. Certainly, the way that most non-disabled people 'talk' about disabled people is often removed from disabled people's conceptualization of disability as a socially created phenomenon. However, as we have seen, it is also true that many disability texts are read from a very narrow perspective and are often taken out of context. Moreover, there has always been a sense in which disability studies preaches to the converted, and it is now the case that 'the converted' are bringing their new and/or different knowledges to disability studies in the form of reflexivity.

We must also stress that disabled people are at different stages in their 'personal and political journeys towards understanding themselves, their material circumstances and their social situations' (Oliver 1996a: 3), and this must provide the context for how we read their stories. Thus, if we take the first section of this book, for example, reading the chapters together yields important information about these stages – each chapter provides a context for all the others – whereas if they are assumed to be self-contained and separate it is easier to diminish them with value judgements and comparisons. For many, the first stage in this understanding, as we have found, is a recognition of shared experiences – both of oppression itself and, later, of collective resistance, because, in Foucault's terms (1972) knowledge is not something that we *have*, but something that we *do*. The first stage of this process cannot happen for many disabled people if personal narratives are confined to or hidden within certain means of expression or certain media – indeed this simply colludes with the culture of 'silence' which is part of disability oppression. And it is also impossible if personal narratives are censored in the interests of homogeneity and reductionism, because it must ultimately only lead to partial political unity (Corker 1998).

## Conclusion

The previous section suggests that the discursive analysis of disability might have much to offer disability studies. To this end, we have brought together a number of international contributors to explore its potential. These contributions reflect the different layers of critical discourse analysis, challenging preconceived 'readings' of texts and stressing the importance of history, politics, hegemony and context, or what discourse analysts sometimes call the 'co-texts' which create particular meanings. However, we have also attempted to go beyond this in giving 'voice' to many of the silenced, 'borderline' or unfamiliar stories of disability studies, for example, the voices of disabled children, disabled women, non-Western perspectives on disability, acquired disability, and cognitive, intellectual, sensory and social disabilities. It is our hope that this will add a considerable body of 'new' knowledges to disability studies, along with alternative ways of theorizing disability and being disabled which will increase the repertoire of resources that disabled people can draw upon in challenging disability oppression.

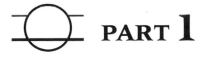 **PART 1**

# PERSONAL NARRATIVES

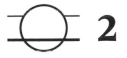 **2**

# Inside aphasia

## Sue Boazman

### Introduction

No one can truly analyse the effects of losing the power of language and communication, for it is a very personal and emotional thing. One can only imagine. I have first-hand experience, for I became aphasic in 1989 following a brain haemorrhage. I have come a long way since that time. I have experienced all sorts of emotional upheavals which continue to affect my life, and those around me, both in a positive and negative way. I soon came to realize that, above all else, the ability to communicate was of paramount importance to me. Perhaps even more so than overcoming my physical disability. With my ability to communicate destroyed, it seemed as if the very core of my personality had been wrenched from me. In retrospect, not being able to express my feelings and emotions verbally was the biggest loss of all, at that time. I felt as if I was at the mercy of all the nursing staff at the hospital, and of well-wishers who came to visit me. With my thought processes still intact, losing my speech was like being locked inside my own head.

Aphasia is a disability that is not instantly recognizable unless you are familiar with it. Because of the complex way speech and language are processed in the brain, many of the associated problems are invisible. The psychological effect can be dramatic. Not only coming to terms with a physical impairment, but also a perceived change in the expressive personality that you once were. Mine was a typical reaction to the loss and grief of this type of trauma. I identify closely with the words of Brumfitt (1985), who wrote: 'people see their past self, before their illness, as very similar to their ideal self, therefore becoming a longed for and yearned for identity'. This sense of loss is often the most difficult to come to terms with, not only to the person with aphasia, but also to the people close to them. Berne also introduced a salient point when he said: 'spontaneity means option, the freedom to choose and express one's feelings' (Berne 1966). From a personal point of view, the ability to be spontaneous is the one thing I miss most of all. Now, I find, my choices and options are limited. Many of the things that I used to do as a matter of course, now require some forethought and preparation beforehand. Aphasia restricts my freedom to express my thoughts and feelings, verbally, and this leads to a feeling of being very much out of control.

Therefore in this chapter, I feel it is important to highlight some of the issues of language and communication that I have come across, as a person who has aphasia. I will attempt to describe the emotional pitfalls that occur, as I carry out what used to be simple everyday tasks, but now require meticulous planning. I will also focus on the attitudes and prejudice that sometimes stand in my way as a person who happens to have a speech disability.

## Controlling communication

Using the telephone is a prime example of the stress and anxiety that can be involved in carrying out such a simple everyday procedure. The situation is made worse if I know that I am going to be speaking to a complete stranger. Before I pick up the receiver, I try to anticipate the conversation. Then I write it all down, making contingency plans in case the conversation does not run according to my expectations. The tone of voice of the person on the other end of the telephone affects my response as well. If the person replies in a friendly and relaxed manner, then I feel relaxed as well. In turn my speech is more fluent. If, on the other hand, the response is offhand and brusque, this affects my speech adversely. I begin to have word-finding difficulties, and my mind goes blank. The more irritated the person on the other end of the telephone becomes, the more I begin to fantasize about how he or she perceives me. I recognize that this, of course, may well be my problem.

I first began to use public transport a few months after my stroke. Using public transport felt risky. I insisted on doing it by myself, because I was desperately trying to regain my independence. I remember one particular incident, which occurred when travelling by bus. Making sure that I had the correct bus fare in my pocket, to avoid the threat of conversation with the driver, I got on the bus. However, when my stop was imminent, there was no bell within reach. I could not stand up while the bus was in motion, for due to the effect of the stroke, I knew I would lose my balance. Due to the noise of the bus, I could not make the driver hear, and we sailed past my stop. I felt rising panic. Another passenger alerted the driver to my plight, but by this time, we had gone a mile down the road. This presented a dual problem. The driver became abusive and started to blame me for not letting him know in time. I tried to explain, but my mind went blank and I was unable to find the right words. It was only when I got up, to get off the bus, that my physical disability became apparent. At this point, the tables turned somewhat and he became covered with confusion and embarrassment. From my point of view, having all the attention focused on me was a nightmare. It drew attention to my aphasia and my disability all at once, and I too became covered with confusion and embarrassment.

These scenarios describe situations where I have been alone to deal with these issues. However, social gatherings can often be very stressful for me, particularly among people I do not know well. While this has always been a problem, even before my stroke, the situation is magnified now because of my aphasia. I am either constantly aware of my speech, or closely watching for a reaction of some kind on the face of the person I am in conversation with. I tend to shy away from conversations that are in danger of becoming too complex. My aphasia is made even worse when I feel under pressure, or when I am tired. Although I am fully aware of this, sometimes there is little I can do to prevent these situations occurring. People who do not recognize the signs, tell me that they are unaware that I am aphasic, but they are oblivious to the inner battle that is continually present inside of me.

In the early days of becoming aphasic, my perception of self changed almost daily. I went through a period of false security, when I was convinced that I would regain perfect speech, although I accepted that my physical capabilities would never be the same. It was only when I began to realize that my speech would be affected for life that I began to go through what I now recognize as the process of mourning. This began to manifest itself in various ways, but mainly through anger, grief and depression. Nurses and therapists bore the brunt of my frustration. My identity had been snatched away, and in its place was a person I no longer recognized. This point is so accurately highlighted by Peggy Dalton (1994):

> The so-called catastrophic reactions which others find difficult to respond to, may be viewed as sudden dilation in the face of confusion. What triggers off the burst of anger or grief or seemingly excessive laughter may in itself seem small. But to the person, the strong emotion may well relate to an awareness of far more than we have perceived from the outside.

Harry Clarke (1996) relates a moving story which occurred when he was first in hospital, recovering from his stroke. He told me:

> When I went into the speech therapy room, I was feeling very frustrated and angry. The therapist started her session, but all I wanted to do was to tell her how I felt. But all that came out of my mouth were unintelligible nonsense. I could feel my anger building, until I could not stand it any longer. Suddenly, I swept everything off of her desk. Pencils, pens, paper, work sheets – the lot! Poor woman, she just sat and gaped at me. Now I had her full attention, and that was all I wanted. Although I knew I wasn't making much sense, the release was immense, and to the lady's credit, she just let me babble on until the end of the session. She didn't interrupt or say a word, and that was the best therapy she could have given me at that time. Afterwards, I had such a sense of relief.

I have two daughters, one aged 10 and the other aged 13. They have grown up with my aphasia and take my speech problems in their stride. As a family, we share a lot of humour together, which certainly helps my situation tremendously. When I had just had my stroke, I remember coming home for the day and my eldest daughter, then 4, brought her 5-year-old friend in to see me. At that time, I was unable to say more than a couple of words, and on seeing the two girls, made an effort to talk to them. They let me mumble on for a bit, and then my daughter said to her friend, 'excuse my strange mother!'. We all thought this was highly amusing, but in reality, my daughter hit the nail on the head when she used the word 'strange'. From her perspective, my speech was strange, and my lop-sided appearance (for I was paralysed on my right side) was indeed strange. To a 4-year-old child, whose whole routine had been disrupted, and whose world had been turned upside down, it was no wonder that she used those amazingly accurate words. Now my eldest daughter is a teenager, who is at the age where arguments with me seem to be an everyday occurrence. Sometimes her arguments are strong and forceful, and it is at times like these that I feel most vulnerable. My speech feels clumsy and incomplete, and I feel very much out of control. Having said that, I am glad that she feels able to do this because she obviously doesn't see my aphasia as any kind of barrier between us, and continues to argue with me regardless!

By comparison, I find that I can function very well in situations where I feel in control. My younger daughter was only 2 years old when I had my stroke, and has never known me to be any different. She too does not see my aphasia as a problem, in fact she will sometimes mimic me and we both laugh together. Because there is no hint of malice, I take it as a compliment that she also feels comfortable enough to do this in my presence. However, in group situations, a different problem materializes. My stroke has altered the volume and pitch of my voice, so that when taking part in group discussions, I sometimes have difficulty making myself heard. I have to wait for an opportunity to break into the conversation before I can get my word in. By the time that happens, the thought I was so desperately trying to hold on to has disappeared. This is a frustration that can be overcome by having the confidence to ask the group to acknowledge my problem. The groups I have worked with in the past have all been willing to respond to my needs. Most importantly, I need the space to talk and put my thoughts in order without interruption.

## Confused discourses

When I first had my stroke, I had to learn to be creative about conveying my needs to others. Being a natural introvert made this especially embarrassing and difficult for me to deal with. With my new 'condition', I had acquired many real and imaginary labels. Overnight, I had become aphasic, disabled, a stroke victim, helpless and dumb. In the hospital, the people that I had the most contact with were nurses, consultants, and therapists of one kind or another. Their response towards me varied greatly. Some showed great compassion, while others showed complete indifference. I had no way of communicating the fact that I was a bright, intelligent, whole human being. This is what hurt the most. Now, eight years after my stroke, the times when I feel under pressure, or have anxious feelings, are still reflected in my speech and language. I know that this is a fact. The difference is that now, I can say with confidence that I am my own expert and I know what my limitations and capabilities are. I would not presume to know the needs of others in a similar situation.

Alarmingly, evidence suggests that this is not always the case among some professionals. In one of her publications, Chris Ireland writes of her own experience of being misdiagnosed as mentally ill. She had in fact suffered a stroke with the added complication of aphasia. This misdiagnosis resulted in her spending time in a mental hospital. While battling to communicate, she was faced with the added problem of prejudice and misunderstanding. She writes:

> Once the consultant saw my notes from the mental hospital, she changed. She became impatient. I tried to write to communicate. Impatiently she told me to put down my notebook, and told me I did not need it. I felt I had lost my only channel of communication with the world.

> (Ireland 1990)

Some elderly people have also had the misfortune to experience this kind of prejudice, and have been wrongly diagnosed as having dementia when in truth, they are aphasic (Rossiter 1990). These stories highlight some of the more exceptional instances of misunderstanding that can occur with aphasia.

I also have personal experience of this kind of prejudice. Having gained a certificate of counselling skills after two years, and been accepted on to the subsequent Diploma course, quite naturally I assumed my path to becoming a counsellor was set. At the point where we were ready to take on our first clients, all students had to take an external assessment and I felt quite confident about this. Unfortunately my interview did not go as I had visualized it. To begin with, the assessor was not expecting to see a disabled person arrive on the doorstep, and looked physically shocked to see me. During the interview, I spoke openly on the subject of my problems with speech and language as a result of my stroke. However, the outcome of the interview was negative. The assessor's report paid direct attention to my word-finding problems. Part of the report read, and I quote:

> my doubts about her working as a psychodynamic counsellor stem from one aspect of her disability, which is her difficulty in finding words. How a client will feel about Sue, who has a speech disability is an important issue.

The emotional damage that this report had on me was catastrophic. In his book, Wilson (1989) describes my feelings most accurately:

From time to time, our self image is liable to be altered uncomfortably by events. 'Life Changes' such as losing a spouse or a job, or failing an important examination, can severely undermine our sense of identity and disorientate us.

My confidence was destroyed from that moment on, and my aphasia worsened considerably. My word finding became appalling, and my momentary memory blocks increased almost immediately. I began to doubt my own ability, and thought long and hard about my decision to become a counsellor. For a while, I had certainly lost my sense of identity, and my self-image was at an all time low. Looking back now, I can see that this was a period of enormous growth for me. Indeed, I learnt more about myself during that time than I did throughout the whole three years on the course. I emerged enriched and strengthened by this painful experience, with my sense of survival complete and intact.

## Conclusion

The implied images of disability in general are often misconstrued and misunderstood. The implied images being that people with disabilities are helpless, dependent and victims, as is illustrated in parts of this chapter. I have also shown that even some professional people demonstrate fixed ideas of what being disabled really means. Carole Pound (1993) suggests that there is a tendency for therapists to focus predominantly on impairment whilst disabled people, not surprisingly, are more aware of the wider social impact of their disability. Aphasia is only recently starting to become recognized as a disability in its own right. It is important, therefore, that some of these issues are highlighted publicly, in order to begin to make headway for the future.

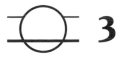 **3**

# The wind gets in my way

## Sally French

### Introduction

Being visually disabled gives rise to many difficulties when attempting to communicate with sighted people. These range from obvious problems, like being unable to recognize people, to more subtle matters like failing to share similar experiences and being unable adequately to describe one's own reality. Conflicting discourses arise when sighted people define what is 'acceptable' and 'normal' behaviour for a visually disabled person and use these definitions to contest that person's identity.

As a small child I had a dislike of going out on windy days. My mother, no doubt exasperated, asked me why this was so, to which I replied 'The wind gets in my way.' I do not remember this incident but it is recalled, as an amusing family story, to show what a quaint and peculiar child I was. As a visually disabled adult I know exactly what I meant. Going out on windy days *is* more difficult. The wind makes a noise which obscures the small auditory cues which, though rarely appreciated until they are absent, are so helpful when walking about. Wearing a hat which covers the ears (as no doubt I did as a child) exacerbates the problem. I was right, the wind does indeed get in my way.

Interpreting the visual world without much sight is difficult, especially for young children who, inevitably, lack experience. Nobody interpreted my fear of walking over zebra crossings correctly, nor my dread of stepping near the edge of flower beds – and yet to me zebra crossings were steps to fall down and flower beds dark, bottomless pits. A common feature of life as a visually disabled person, which starts very early, is having constantly to explain oneself and yet rarely having one's experiences confirmed. There were other behaviours which I knew were sensible but which I had no words to explain. 'Not looking where I was going' was one. It seemed particularly perverse to the adults in my life that, as a visually disabled child, I constantly looked at the ground! What is more, I always trailed behind out of everybody's sight. As a visually disabled adult, however, I have no difficulty explaining these 'aberrant' behaviours. The ground is where most of the danger lies; by looking down I have the greatest likelihood of seeing objects or steps in my path. True I sometimes get slapped in the face by an overgrown hedge, but ground objects are far more common and my distance vision is so restricted that looking down is much more functional than looking up. As for lagging behind, well, following other people, looking at what they do, observing their feet to see where they tread, is a sensible way to behave. It is they, not I, who are finding the steps, it is they who are finding the way.

How often these conflicting exchanges occurred I cannot say, but I can still experience the feelings they induced; feelings of isolation, difference and shame. The feelings were made worse by my inability to explain my behaviour, even to myself, although I always knew that I was right and 'they' were wrong. Experiences such as these had an adverse effect on my self-esteem and confidence which only began to abate when, in an abusive boarding school at the age of nine, I met other girls like me. Living our lives together, having them as my friends and knowing they shared my world was nothing short of joy. These deeply rooted friendships are still important; they have buffered my life.

## Communication in a sighted world

It is estimated that most communication between people occurs at the non-verbal level, and that if verbal and non-verbal behaviours conflict people tend to believe the non-verbal messages as they are far more difficult to conceal or control. Visually disabled people, to varying degrees, do not have access to non-verbal communication and must rely much more heavily on what is actually said. Exceptions to this are the non-verbal qualities of voice (pitch, tone, speed, volume and so on), where much information about the person's emotional state can be gauged, and touch – which social norms largely prohibit outside intimate social and sexual contexts. As visually disabled people we tend to lose the emotional content of messages, though the non-verbal qualities of voice, and even the sound of someone walking, or shuffling in a chair, can give a great deal of information.

It is difficult for us, particularly in group situations, to assess people's attitudes and moods because of the lack of non-verbal information. If I make a comment in a meeting, for example, I am frequently unaware how the comment has been received especially if nobody answers me directly; whether they are smiling and nodding, or looking angry or bored are beyond my perceptions. Neither can I see if people look tired or unwell. Non-verbal communication is largely learnt, so our own non-verbal behaviour may be reduced or different from that of sighted people – I have variously been told that my non-verbal communication is 'impoverished' and 'no different' from that of others. Lack of non-verbal behaviour can disturb interaction, particularly in group situations and where visual disability is not understood or accepted. It is, for example, very difficult to contribute to group discussion without interrupting people as 'turn taking' is governed by subtle visual cues – something I only learnt through studying psychology. This can cause hostility in others and embarrassment in ourselves and can lead us to remain silent.

Noisy, crowded environments are particularly difficult. The background noise obscures the voice, which cannot be compensated with non-verbal communication. It also obliterates the auditory cues that we use to orientate ourselves and to move around. Communication in noisy environments often demands the use of both verbal and non-verbal communication. Visually disabled people cannot, for example, hear speech when sitting opposite someone in a train because of the inability to supplement the voice with non-verbal information such as that gained from lip reading. When I am lecturing to large groups of students I cannot hear their questions, not because I am deaf, but because I cannot supplement what I hear with what I see. Neither can I make eye contact with the person who is speaking.

An example from my own experience, which illustrates the importance of non-verbal communication, occurred when I gave a 'one-off' guest lecture to a group of students who were undertaking a health service management course. When the course leader sent me the students' evaluation of my performance I was shocked to discover how bad it was – in my 15 years of teaching I had never received such a negative judgement. The students had found me 'distant', 'cold', 'aloof' and 'uninterested'. Admittedly I was tired, but I was well prepared and delivered what I thought was an interesting session. I certainly did not feel any of the emotions with which I was credited. So what could be wrong?

There was only one obvious difference between this lecture and the many hundreds I had given before: I had not explained my visual disability. Usually I tell students that I cannot see them as individuals and that none of their non-verbal language will reach me. I encourage them to speak up and never to be afraid of interrupting me. But this time I had failed to do so. As someone who has been visually disabled from birth, it is difficult for me to judge the impact which distorted non-verbal communication might have on a sighted audience, but most people to whom I have related this story are convinced that the problem lay entirely with my lack of explanation of visual disability. The likelihood of visual disability rarely features in people's interpretations of our behaviour; instead we are credited with negative personal characteristics.

White sticks can be used to supplement communication. I use a white stick intermittently as a symbol of visual disability. I use it to influence people's behaviour, for example to attract their help or alert them to take care. Often the symbolism of the white stick supplements verbal information. When I want help to find a building, for example, saying 'I can't see very well', with a white stick displayed, gives a more powerful message than saying the same words without a white stick. The white stick is not, however, powerful enough to prevent people giving visual directions both verbally and non-verbally – much to their own embarrassment. Although some people are better than others, I find it best to ask directions of other visually disabled people who will provide me with appropriate non-visual and near-visual cues. Saying 'turn left when you get to the rusty gate' is likely, for example, to be far more helpful than saying 'turn left when you get to the police station'. Contrary to biblical predictions the blind can lead the blind and it is very unlikely that either will fall in the ditch!

I have used a white stick for 30 years and have noticed a change in people's responses especially in recent times. It used to be the case that people assumed total blindness, but now the question 'are you partial?' is common. Similarly, if I am treated as a totally blind person and I say 'I can see a bit' this does not give rise to surprise. Despite this, I do not feel that people will understand or believe if, having used a white stick to cross a busy road, I fold it up and read a book. The feeling of discomfort to which this gives rise in the presence of others is very strong, although I have rarely been challenged.

Such a challenge did, however, occur a few months ago. I was meeting a friend for lunch on a very busy street. The pavement was crowded so I used my white stick to avoid bumping into people as I walked along. Being rather early for my appointment I folded the stick and went into a shop to browse around the books. I was approached by a middle-aged woman who, having seen me in both situations, challenged my behaviour with some hostility. I gave a terse, rather angry, explanation to which she replied, with a very mild voice, that she had not understood but that now she did.

Occasionally people (usually old people) ask questions such as 'How long have you been like this?' or want explanations of cause. Others find it hard to believe that only a small amount of help is required. The question 'Which road am I in?', for example, is frequently followed by the question 'Where do you want to go?' Others seem to equate visual disability with illness and dependency. I was recently told by someone who was helping me to find the entrance to a railway station that it was a good job he worked for the Red Cross and another was incensed that 'people like me' were compelled to work. On a recent occasion, when using a white stick in the council buildings, I was told 'You're going the wrong way, you need the Social Services Department'!

Responses such as these are, however, relatively rare, especially in recent times. Most people I approach are willing to help in any way they can and many volunteer. Mostly I am treated with respect. Taking control by stating, with assurance, exactly what help is needed seems to discourage condescension and patronage and induce relaxation and confidence in those whose help is sought.

My feelings about using a white stick are mixed. I regard it as a symbol of independence rather than a symbol of dependency. It is understood throughout the world and has assisted me in travelling with confidence to unfamiliar countries on my own. I constantly feel, however, that others are judging me and thinking I am a fraud, though this is rarely voiced and may not be the case. I am reluctant to use the white stick in the vicinity of sighted people I know, for fear of what I think might be their judgement. I feel, but do not believe, that, as someone who can see (albeit minimally) I should not be using it.

These perceptions of what other people think were reinforced in a recent *Songs of Praise* television programme which came from Exeter Cathedral. One of the people interviewed was an instructor from the training centre of the Guide Dogs for the Blind Association in the city. He explained how he, as a sighted person, worked the dogs, as a blind person would, to ensure their competence and safety. He went on to say that he always identified himself as a trainer, if people tried to help him, as he thought it would be detrimental to visually disabled people if the public thought he was visually disabled and subsequently saw him looking in a shop window. The message, that visually disabled people who use aids, and yet can see, are frauds, was broadcast to the nation even though the Guide Dogs for the Blind Association actively encourage people with my degree of vision to apply for training.

## Contesting and confirming our identities

Our attempts at communicating within a sighted world give rise to isolation and lack of acceptance by sighted people. I do not think I would ever be described as an isolated person, neither would I describe myself in that way – I have many good friends, I have relatives, I have work colleagues, I go on holiday to exciting places with other people – and yet visual disability is, for me, in some situations at least, an isolating experience. This is largely due to my inability to recognize people and to see and respond to non-verbal language. It is also due to other people's lack of understanding and acceptance of visual disability and their lack of adaptation to it.

I have lived in the same house for 16 years and yet I cannot recognize my neighbours. I know nothing about them at all; which children belong to whom, who has come and gone, who is old or young, ill or well, black or white. When I had a painter in recently he told me more about the 'goings on' in my road than I could ever know. I am a lecturer and yet I cannot recognize my students. I explain the situation and we work together well but I cannot greet them, smile at them, give them a friendly wave, and I cannot receive their gestures in return. I work within a bustling, vibrant environment and yet I often feel detached. I am surrounded by people, some of whom say 'Hello', but I rarely know who they are.

On occasions I have made efforts to find solutions to problems such as these. On moving to my present house I informed several neighbours that, because of my inability to recognize them, I would doubtless pass them by in the street without greeting them. One neighbour, who had previously seen me striding confidently down the road, refused to believe me, but the others said they understood and would talk to me if our paths crossed. For the first couple of weeks it worked and I was surprised how often we met, but after that their greetings rapidly decreased and then ceased altogether. Why this happened I am not sure, but I suspect that my lack of recognition strained the interaction and limited the social reward they received from the encounter. For my part, my inability to see them approaching meant that I was invariably jolted abruptly from my thoughts when they did speak which, as well as feeling unpleasant, affected the normality of my response.

My neighbours were presented with a learning opportunity to which they initially responded but then declined. If they had persisted it is likely that the difficulties would have diminished; I would have recognized their voices and getting to know each other better would have reduced the tension we all experienced. Simply informing people about visual disability is seldom enough to change significantly their behaviour.

In 1996, when on holiday in Greenland with a friend, Daisy, who is totally blind, I did, however, have a very different experience. We were to join a group of 15 people and would take part in various outdoor activities. Precise information was difficult to get, the tour operator said that he had never had any visually disabled tourists going to Greenland before but that the Greenlanders were 'very friendly'. He was optimistic, but when questioned closely about possible difficulties, would not commit himself. The holiday was expensive but, drawing on each other's strength, we booked it up.

On the first day we went on a long, but easy, walk. Daisy held a white stick most of the time. I guided Daisy but displayed a white stick on several occasions to attract help for myself, for example when boarding a boat. The other people on the tour willingly gave their help, though their interaction with us was tentative and shy. By the second day I realized that they must have been observing us closely to understand our situation. From that day on their help was spontaneous and absolutely right. When things became difficult we both had a guide, but as soon as we could manage their help was appropriately withdrawn. The pace of the holiday was slow and we were given opportunities to experience things in our own way. The boat was steered near an iceberg so that Daisy could feel its length, I was always ensured the best position to see, and the other tourists, even with minimal English, described to us what they saw. We felt totally relaxed and did not use a white stick for the remainder of the holiday. This experience has led to a marked shift in my judgement of the capacity of sighted people to comprehend the complexities of visual disability. When we returned home I rang the tour operator to tell of our success. He was, of course, delighted, and said that people who visited Greenland were 'not your average tourist'. Their response was certainly very different from that of my neighbours.

Being with sighted people can be a very relaxing experience in some respects; they can find the way, lead us around, drive us in cars, but our different experiences of the world can threaten the enjoyment of our interactions. A few years ago I went on holiday to the Channel Islands with a visually disabled friend. She had always been on holiday with sighted people before but, although we were restricted and had many hassles resulting from visual disability, she claimed that the holiday had been more enjoyable and successful than any other she had had.

We cannot always engage in the same activities as sighted people, we cannot do things as fast, we need more time to see, and we need opportunities to use our other senses to the full. When we are together, getting lost and having problems, we are *engaging* with the world far more than we ever could from a car or at someone else's pace. We might not do as much, but what we do is on *our* terms and at *our* pace and without any need to explain ourselves. It is difficult, when with sighted people, to meet our own needs without curtailing theirs and it is easy for relationships to become unequal leading to feelings of isolation, injustice and boredom. The behaviour of the people on the Greenland trip was sophisticated; they gave us the help we needed, they helped us to experience things on our own terms, while at the same time respecting our capabilities, autonomy and independence.

## Conclusion

Visual disability has a profound effect on communication, not only in terms of everyday interaction, but in terms of what we know, what we experience, how we behave and who we are. The aids that we use – white sticks, monoculars, guide dogs – also have a profound effect on how we feel, how we behave and how others respond to us. When groups of visually disabled people come together the 'rules' of social discourse are changed. People may, for example, shout out somebody's name in order to find that person, or walk around uninhibited where the act of bumping into someone and asking 'Who are you?' solves the problem of recognition. We have our own humour, and a unique history of 'special' schools, 'special' colleges, 'special' equipment, 'special' jobs and 'special' ways of doing things. Perhaps this indicates the existence of a 'blind culture' where, in a similar way to 'Deaf culture', social rules and behaviour take on a specific form to overcome social barriers and where, despite our great diversity, common experiences in our past and present lives bind us together in so many ways.

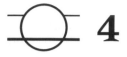

# 4

# I am more than my wheels

## Sandy Slack

### Introduction

> I wonder if I've been changed in the night? Let me think: was I the same when I got up this morning? I almost think I can remember feeling a little different. But if I'm not the same, the next question is, 'Who in the world am I?' Ah, that's the great puzzle.
>
> (Lewis Carroll, *Alice in Wonderland*)

The above quotation has cropped up in my life on very significant occasions with uncanny regularity. The consistent theme has always been amidst a change in my life. The first time I recalled the words was during trauma and confusion when I realized my life as I knew it would never be the same as yesterday. The 'puzzle' represented the alien responses of others towards me. On another occasion I was reassured because I realized the words took on a different meaning and their interpretation became one of inspiration and hope. I used the quotation during an exercise with a group when the theme was one of personal growth, renewal and positive change. In the latter the 'puzzle' was removed and replaced with an integrated self which had chosen and welcomed change. In this sense I have very little puzzle about who I am, but I am more puzzled by what others perceive me to be.

It is a reminder that words are only of their time and place. Transpose them to another time and place and they can take on a whole new meaning. So it was I learnt that all those words gathered in the school playground which seemed harmless in a simple sense echoed back to me in memory with most painful force. Words like 'cripple', 'spas', 'mental', stupid', 'clumsy' 'blind as a bat', and 'deaf as a post'. I could go on, but even reviving and actually writing these words feels abusive. I suspect there is no culture in the world which has not used words to further disable disabled people. If this is the global diet no wonder disabled people have struggled all this time not with the actuality of their impairment, not just the history of labelling and segregation, but the representation placed in people's minds of what constitutes a disabled person. The agenda has been set since time began and finds its many roots in biblical terms like the relationship of sin and suffering to disability and disease. Two phrases come to mind, delivered by a one-time friend: 'of course the experience of suffering makes you a stronger person' and 'God only gives you as much as he thinks you can bear.' To the first I ask why is it that there are thousands of people who I would call strong who have managed to avoid the 'suffering trip'? To the second, God never asked me what my tolerance level for suffering is and if he had he would maybe change his mind if he was truly into this thing called compassion.

'Who in the world am I?' was likened to a record jammed in the same groove playing the same piece over and over in my head. Being me in a changed image almost became unbearable. Except the image did not belong to me. It was created by the external world as if it wanted to obliterate the original version of me. My unique pattern was redundant – surplus to requirement. The past was irrelevant. Never mind that my spirit – my very essence – thrived on physical expression. My relationship to the world and the thing which gave it meaning was translated through the physical. Therein lies a complexity. The external world set up a new plate and printed me onto their headed paper for all to recognize should they need too. My internal world was imprisoned with all this unexpressed movement. I had lost my dominant language and had not yet learnt the new one.

## Before

The transition into a wheelchair user from a physical education teacher who thrived on space and freedom and movement was not easy. For a start no one told me what I should do with all this store of anger which grew into volcanic proportions inside of me. I was so frightened of all that anger. How could such volume be contained safely inside one body and never seep to escape causing unsuspecting harm? Just like the nuclear reactors scattered across our world. Such power has to go somewhere – doesn't it?

The language I knew and felt so at ease with is no longer accessible to me. My language was the one of movement. The sheer heaven and joy of expression through movement gave me all the language I thought I would ever need.

A triangle is formed between the thumb and index finger and they rest in total tension on the white line; there is silence and utter stillness; the tummy flutters and the adrenalin is stored to capacity in the body ready for the optimum moment. The gun fires. There is only one aim and that is to reach that line as fast as possible and break the tape before anyone else. Victory is sweet but transient. The very act of running at speed is sweeter. The harmony of blending this journey together and the unique noise of spikes piercing the cinder track was sensuous. I could be the only person in the world at that moment – almost flying in the wind. Utter bliss. I wonder if modern athletes feel the same with all their pressures to win and earn money? They must have started out with that sense of joy and physical completeness.

I recall the thrill of sprinting towards the high box. I knew how to place my hands on the box at the exact moment which would take my body high into the air. My legs thrust and my hips circle my body and then release moving through the air unsupported in the certain knowledge I would land on the other side. Total control and yet a second of pure freedom from gravity.

The challenge of the moving rope, timing the connection with it precisely, swinging through the air as one; turning around it drawing pictures in the air and then letting go as the shared moment ended.

Sunny October mornings, fresh dewed grass, whisper of smoky breath circling the frosty air were moments to cherish. You know you will spend the next hour and a half or so criss-crossing that turf working with a team, using your skill towards a common end. Clicking of sticks, voices muttering when it goes badly, screeches and exhilaration if you manage to score. The anticipation of this shared experience was more than a game. It felt like an expression of who I was and encompassed my talents, my skills, my spirit and my love of comradeship. Being with and trusting others.

Gymnastics, dance, athletics, swimming, team games – they are more than the surface observation. To those who take part they are a language. They require focused concentration, skill and knowledge, but all these without the internal spirit which drives you forward are meaningless. To use the body to its maximum capabilities is like painting that picture or writing that book or playing that music – it is almost spiritual. That was my language. I communicated with the world and myself through the medium of perpetual motion. It was who I was.

## After

Is it really so long ago and yet acutely present in the memory? I have now been a disabled person almost as long as I was a non-disabled person. I often ask myself if I am two personalities – before and after? Or am I an integrated person blending my first 29 years of life into the last 23 years? What would I be like if I had not been injured? Then of course one has to allow for ordinary self-development which is coloured by all kinds of life events over the years. I suspect I would be much the same inherently, but much less informed about the variety of lifestyles people choose or have forced upon them. I would perhaps be more complacent and take ordinary things for granted if I hadn't experienced this added dimension in my life. I would have missed out on meeting some amazing people committed to ensuring rights for disabled people. I would certainly be more financially secure but would I be any happier?

I have read the books. I have assimilated the theory. I have shared all this with others informally and formally. I have invited others to view the world

in a different way in the hope of accommodating difference into a more harmonious world. I have done all this and continue to do this because I am
always hopeful that people's capacity for change is infinite. This is what I
believe. When my belief is tested out in reality – when I look at the facts in the
cold light of day – I could be forgiven for wavering from my original belief.
What I choose to share with you I hope will resemble my belief and my
uncertainty. You will find both present. I offer no neat and tidy answers to the
challenges which face disabled people who find themselves in a society
which purports to empower and in spite of good intentions manages to
disempower.

## Miscommunication

Communication from where I am sitting is not straightforward. It gets tricky
and complicated. I think it may be because two languages are operating. What
I am seeing is different from what non-disabled people see. We are coming
from separate reference points and often move in a different direction. I may
see the mountain and they may see a hump. I long to glide and wheel in harmony with my environment. These are the moments when I feel who I am
and can be in touch with my physical and emotional self prior to being disabled. These moments of freedom are my truth.

I always feel alone with my frustration. Here a complex set of feelings come
into play. Most friends deny me my justified anger, and because of their
embarrassment I am drawn into a game which on the one hand wants to protect them but on the other hand scream at them for not seeing the oppression
for what it is. When some friends adopt the tight-lipped silent approach I can
hear their silent voice saying 'here she goes again'. I infrequently hear them
say they understand and can see the oppression and support my protest. The
worst is when they move into the parent voice with 'never mind we must
make the best of it'. I scream inside at the patronizing tones.

If only people could see anger as a positive force for change instead of an
ugly creature best not talked about I believe we would achieve better results.
I sense I am touching on a British culture issue here and already can feel the
offence it may cause with some readers! This is part of the complexity. Having
the oppression acknowledged at the time feels really empowering – so people
who seek to find ways of empowering disabled people here is a start!

When well-meaning people respond with 'you should write to them about
it', I am then deemed responsible for all the changes which need to happen in
order to access ordinary things. If I spent my time writing to 'them' I would
have little time or energy left to earn a living or socialize. Yet I am left thinking
if I don't write they won't either and the barrier will never be removed. I have
to reach a compromise by writing about some things and letting others go by.
I try to encourage non-disabled people to take responsibility but with a few
exceptions they do not feel it is anything to do with them. Not yet in their life
anyway.

I have to stay firm in the knowledge of who I am and not be deflected by the constant barrage of other people's miscommunications. Sometimes it feels like words are just thrown at me and I am expected to field them in an intelligent way. I could fill a chapter with examples! Here are some: Stranger, 'were you born like that?'; 'what do you do all day?'; 'you work – aren't you marvellous!'; 'I will put you over there ... [not where would you like to be]'; 'It's good there is an adapted toilet for people like you, isn't it?' These are just a snippet of usual comments from strangers. From some friends they get worse. I say worse because friends have knowledge of you beyond the wheelchair but when pushed have a curious habit of colluding with non-disabled people. I think it must be about 'mustn't make a fuss ...' On being oppressed verbally and barrier-wise at the theatre, friend's response – tight-lipped silence. I am on my island again – alone. Similar occasion, 'never mind look at the beautiful surroundings'. My oppression is blanked the debate is closed. This is a very powerful way of patronizing disabled people and establishes the non-disabled person as the one in control. My oppression is not even important enough to invite discussion. I scream inside. Honest expression of my feelings has been denied.

I think and feel oppression in any form should be the concern of everybody. The reality tells me that people mostly settle for the status quo. I believe if you are not for it you are against it. There is no middle ground because middle ground means do nothing and if nothing is done you are actively supporting the status quo. Translated into disability issues: if access is not available and people accept that is the way it is, they are actively saying they don't want change. They are actively saying it's OK for disabled people to be denied access.

So what with being denied anger, being patronized, protecting friends, taking responsibility for all the barrier issues disabled people face, bringing about the changes required, ordinary life can feel very stressful at times. When I am feeling strong my best ally is my sense of humour. I have a good laugh at myself and the world and gobble up the cruel comments and spit them out. For a time I am free again. The other side of this complicated coin manifests itself in the gratitude game. Many disabled people are so relieved when they don't need to activate the 'fight'/frustration button that they end up saying 'thank you' in an affected manner for something which should be a right in the first place. When did you last hear a non-disabled person get excited about a public toilet which they could use? Or the thrill of seeing automatic doors and a lift in the building?

From day one I have eaten a diet of goodwill, well meaning, persuasion, steady debate until I feel obese with it all. Overflowing with too much trying, bloated with patronage, engorged with the rigidity of the world around me. In the early days it seemed easier to let people do what they needed to do in order to feel good about themselves and confirm my disability. I colluded with this script for a while in an attempt to keep the peace and conserve energy. Until one day with almost thundering realization it dawned on me that this compliance had very little to do with my legs not working or the pain

I experience but everything to do with denying me my rights. My right to move freely and choose a variety of life experiences. That is when the trouble started! I realized that was the point of no return and that I could never again collude with the status quo.

The more I tried to extend my boundaries the more I came across the obstacles. Communication with new people can never be fresh and barrier free, because they draw on their visual sense first and take the cue from there. They have made some judgements already because they are privy to visual information about me which they then feel at liberty to comment on. The opening to the conversation will mostly be, 'how long have you been in a wheelchair?', or 'what happened to you?' Some people think they have a natural right to hear my life story, whether I wish to tell it or not. This poses serious difficulties in a new acquaintance because the agenda for the conversation has been pre-written by someone else. The effect is to block the possibility of opening the conversation with equal information sharing about each other. Non-disabled people would be unlikely to start a conversation with another person by asking them their medical history or about any trauma in their life. It just doesn't work that way. In my wicked moments I want to respond in absurd ways! For example, in reply to how long I have been in the wheelchair, 'since this morning when I fell out of bed!' Or in response to what happened to me, 'now which part of my life would you like – so many things have happened to me – how about you?' I just grow tired and bored with the same gambit.

On a serious level of course the person asking for private information is patronizing and usually has a hidden message in their head saying 'I am glad it's not me.' Or they focus on me to disguise their underlying embarrassment. Some people thrive on focusing on the other person in quite a detailed way because it blocks the necessity for disclosure on their part. It gives an unequal start to the communication by demanding disclosure before an ordinary connection can be made. I wish I could say I have dealt with this dilemma but alas I have not. My responses are as varied as the colours in the rainbow and depend on so many other factors. I am not at all consistent. It depends on who the person is, the occasion, the importance, my mood, my energy, my quickness of mind and my desire not to sound rude on a first meeting. What I wish for the most is that non-disabled people avoid constantly putting me in this position and just for once ask me who I am, or what I do or where I live. A person once said to me 'they are only being friendly . . .', well that is a cop out and does not hold water any longer.

There is an essential difference between showing interest in a person and a desire to satisfy your own insatiable curiosity. The latter shows disregard for boundaries and limits of privacy. The privacy accorded to non-disabled people is often denied to disabled people. The rules change – but not by consensus.

## Wheels as property, symbol or freedom? Learning a new language

I have to get on and learn this new language. 'Have wheels will travel' as the saying goes . . . but there are wheels and there are wheels.

The National Health Service (NHS) developed the first set of self-wheel wheelchairs during the war. War is always an incentive to react differently because values change, agendas change. The war-wounded young men needed a form of transport when they returned home minus bits of the anatomy which were previously essential as a soldier. So the chairs were created and issued free to those who required them. They still issue more or less the same model and occasionally change the paint work – like red instead of grey. They are functional, they are heavy and they are all much the same except for size. Most have labels stuck on them saying they are NHS property.

Property is an interesting word. People who own property see the declaration of it as status. Status usually denotes a positive aspect of a person's standing in the world. It is thought to be insulting to describe a person as property. Married men in Victorian times referred to their wives as part of their property, part of their estate. Of course some men still do this but they are more likely to be challenged if found to hold this view. Disabled people frequently become the property of many authorities. Except this is not a positive status, it is an official statement which can mean you need someone or something in order to live your life. The creation of dependency begins with this process. It has little to do with choice and much to do with how structures are organized. Disabled people variously become 'clients', 'patients' or 'service users'. They are then filed on computer (permission for this practice is rarely sought), and they 'belong' to that department. Disabled people became property in order to beget property.

So what is this property disabled people often need? Well I have noticed that most people who are in work live some distance from their workplace. They are not able to walk the long distance so they usually look for some form of transport for their mobility needs. It may be a private car or public transport. This is considered the norm and in no way would it ever be described as a special need. Disabled people who require a wheelchair or a car for their mobility needs are described as having a special need. To disabled people this is neither need or special, it is an essential norm. Why then is it so difficult to obtain the mobility which is appropriate to that person's life? Why is it that disabled people who cannot walk are told that they must have an NHS wheelchair whether it meets their requirements or not? I think this is structural abuse. I think the whole system is abusive and degrading. Mobility for non-walkers should be a right and the choice of aid should be entirely with the disabled person. A society which holds non-walkers to ransom with outdated equipment not only sends a message of less worth to disabled people but describes the kind of society which is prepared to collude with this abuse. Communicating with a world whose dependency creation builds professional empires and renders disabled people unequal is not a good starting point. It is not a two-way process. Imagine spending hours walking in ill-fitting shoes which cause you pain and difficulty because your fit is not made available!

Of course there are splendid wheelchair designs available now across the world but at a price. They are marketed in glossy brochures as if they were designer items used as accessories not essentials. The whole mobility aid market is offensive because it makes huge profits out of other people's disabilities. The government of course has allowed this to be the case because of its worship of market forces. If the government is to continue with this market force approach then they must make real money available to disabled people so that they may go out and purchase these necessities. No man, woman or child should be confined to their own four walls simply because they cannot afford a suitable mobility aid. We have the technology; we should also have the commitment to exploit it to the full and with pride so all disabled people can live their lives in freedom of movement. Wheelchairs need to be a symbol of freedom not confinement. They are an alternative to walking and provide independence for their users. My wheelchair is my best friend – I wheel it with pride and confidence. It takes me into the world.

Then I am reminded of another structural reality alas. The wheelchair is not 'mine' at all, it is government property. I struggled for years to obtain a job after re-training in a new profession; 11 years to be precise. Of course during that time I lived on benefit, which made buying a suitable wheelchair difficult.

For years I struggled with an NHS model which was heavy especially to get in and out of my car. My health suffered as a result of this struggle and I had increasing pain in my neck, shoulders and arms. This is an example of how disability can be individualized. The outcome of using poor equipment was attributed to my impairment – the deterioration in my health – not to the heaviness of the equipment.

I finally became employed. The government will provide equipment to people in work who are disabled to enable them to function to capacity. Of course you have to agree to register as a disabled person first; you are then issued with a green card confirming you are disabled. Imagine car drivers having to state their inability to walk the distance to work before they were allowed to obtain a car and confirm their walking restriction! Most people would be insulted at such an idea. However that is how it is and this registration is then followed by an assessment whereby an 'expert' decides what might be suitable for you. I wonder where these 'experts' gain their expertise?

I went through the necessary hoops and became the proud recipient of a light-weight wheelchair. I could not believe the difference it made to my life. I wheeled with less effort and pulled the chair into my car so easily and gloried in the paint work which was the colour of my choosing. I felt different. I felt very able. This feeling has continued – until an unpleasant encounter recently with the issuing government agency. I needed to ring them about a small repair – a faulty inner tube which had been missed during a recent service inspection. I paid my local cycle shop to do the repair rather than drive

65 miles to the suppliers saving time and money. The agency, on hearing that my puncture happened during a visit to the theatre, reprimanded me and said I was not expected to use the chair other than when I was working and they could not pay for the repair. I was genuinely shocked at this response and was reminded about government control over disabled people's lives.

A wheelchair is not something you take off at the end of the day! Am I now expected to stay housebound and trapped except when I am working? This demonstrates to me the government's narrow thinking and understanding of a disabled person's lifestyle. Take for example a situation in a work environment: it is Friday and it has been a long week, a colleague suggests we go to the pub for a drink and snack and unwind from the day. This must be a frequent occurrence across the country. However I am not allowed to socialize in my wheelchair! Must I go home, transfer into an old NHS model which is heavy to wheel, heavy to get into the car and looks less attractive and meet the group later, or turn down the offer and go home to social death? What would you do? I must add I already experience social death frequently because of inaccessible buildings and the inaccessible homes of my friends.

You will notice that the personal, public and political faces of disability are revealed. The relationship between the three is not in doubt. However, there will be many who feel and think that disability is only political and indeed it is important and needs to stay in that arena in order for fundamental changes to take place. I subscribe to that view but not exclusively. I think the experience of disability is far more complex and is an interrelated mixture of all three considerations. My continuing challenge is to find a place in this world which is mine as of right not of favour. I still find the human spirit to be quite remarkable. I redefined my image and rejected the one offered to me. I found my own space and continue to work on my freedom. I am still frightened of the anger but have a better understanding of its dynamic.

To deny the individual experience is to deny the human expression of a reality which faces disabled people every day of their lives. There is the internal self and the external self – that applies to all human beings. It is no different for disabled people. The difference as I understand it lies with the power of external factors to influence the internal to such an extent it becomes hard to reconcile the two into a workable harmonious form. It also feels important that the personal and unique history of each disabled person is not disregarded. It forms part of their life script and informs their responses to the disabling barriers they encounter. This is why disabled people are not a 'group' as society would have you believe. Diversity of culture, ethnic origin, religious belief, sexual orientation all form essential differences; although disability is to be found within and across this diversity and can be described as a common factor it does not unite or make 'the same as'.

For each 'group' described there will always be an individual who can tell their story in a different way. The labels gathered along the way, like elderly, disabled, single parent, homeless, lesbian or gay, criminal, disturbed child will all have behind them individuals with a personal experience which does not fit the frame of what constitutes that label in the public eye or the public perception of that label. Each story, each experience is valid and incredibly important if we are to understand what lies behind the label. If each story helps us to change the way we do things then of itself it is invaluable. For too long we have worked in formulas and categories and have failed to hear the story which is born of reality. The more people tell their story the more society will see for themselves where the barriers to living lie. They are so obvious they cannot be missed.

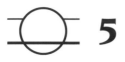 **5**

# Depressed and disabled: some discursive problems with mental illness

## Susan Gabel

### Introduction

In this chapter I explore some discursive problems with the use of the term 'mental illness' by presenting an alternative approach to some arguments and problems of discourse about mental illness. I offer a philosophical rather than an empirical critique of discourses of mental illness and while doing so, I draw upon my own experiences as a person who lives with depression. In this chapter I illustrate two problems within disability discourses which can be illuminated by using the example of mental illness. First, we have long focused on physicality – the assumption that 'disabled-ness' is primarily related to how we appear to others (I will come back to the term 'disabled-ness' below). If we look disabled, we are likely to be perceived as disabled and to feel disabled. If we do not look disabled we are less likely to be perceived as disabled and to feel disabled. I argue that this is not necessarily the case and it should not be the primary way we describe and interpret disabled identity. For example, I do not appear disabled yet I struggle daily as I live a disabled life. On the other hand, I have known individuals who appear significantly disabled to others who do not view themselves as disabled. This should not be surprising if we interpret experiences, including disabled experiences, using the framework proposed within this chapter.

A second problematic discourse in disability studies has been the notion that disability is a social construct (Mehan *et al*. 1986; Lane 1992; Bogdan and Taylor 1994; Trent 1995). The risk of a constructivist framework for understanding disability, and therefore its narrowness, is in its tendency to conceptualize the social construction of disability as *happening to* disabled people rather than *controlled by* them. By this I mean that constructivist theories too often place disabled people in the role of social victim (Gabel 1993, 1994;

King 1993) or as members of a social group oppressed by the able-bodied, or as stigmatized individuals (Bogdan and Biklen 1977; Fine and Asch 1988; Hahn 1988). I am not, however, arguing against a constructivist approach to disability theory. Rather, I am aiming for a different focus within constructivism, one in which the disabled individual herself becomes the active creator of meaning and identity.

As an experiment, let us broadly conceptualize discourse as the construction of meaning, experience as the impetus for discourse, and the body as the medium through which discourse flows through experience to meaning. Within that conceptual framework, imagine any experience of disability, which of necessity is an experience of the body. If the person having the experience concludes that she is disabled, then she is, indeed, disabled. Contrastingly, if the person having the experience concludes that she is not disabled, then she is not disabled. Both conclusions would hold whether or not others observe the disabled-ness and whether or not they agree. In the remainder of this chapter I will elaborate upon these ideas, first by describing my experiences with depression and later by analysing three concepts central to this interpretation of disability; body, experience and being.

## Mental illness

Seven years ago I was diagnosed with double depression. Double depression is a psychiatric diagnosis assigned when an individual experiences chronic mild depression combined with periodic episodes of major depression. At the time of my diagnosis I was experiencing a major depression. Since my diagnosis, I have taken an anti-depressant on a daily basis and I have learnt how to 'manage' my condition so that I live optimally. I know the importance of rest and the way the lack of rest affects my mood. I can recognize the symptoms of inadequate levels of medication. I frequently analyse my thought processes and my relationships to gauge the impact of my condition on myself and others with whom I interact. I do not currently see a therapist, although I have in the past and probably will in the future, since therapy helps me stay cognitively alert to my depression and its consequences.

To the outside world, particularly to individuals with whom I do not live, I appear able-bodied. I have what is often called an 'invisible disability'. It is not usually recognized by others, and when friends or colleagues learn that I have depression and that I view myself as disabled, they usually are surprised. A typical reaction when an acquaintance discovers that I live with depression and that I view myself as disabled is to say, 'You don't look disabled', or 'How can you tell you are depressed?' or 'Is depression a disability?' Nevertheless, I am disabled. I live the life of a disabled person, albeit an invisible disabled person. I am a gimp, at least in a metaphoric sense. My medication is my wheelchair and rest is my access ramp, or perhaps it is the other way round. I am disabled. But am I mentally ill?

Mental illness does not always feel mental nor is it always an illness. When I am depressed, my whole body feels the depression, not just my mind. I feel like my legs and arms are made of lead. I drag my body around, struggling to climb stairs or go for a short walk. I weep unexpectedly, then my eyelids swell and my eyes turn red. I want to sleep endlessly and in sleeping too much, my brain feels foggy and my thinking gets sluggish. I become uninterested in most sensual pleasures. I overeat. I overreact. I misunderstand. Since these experiences occur infrequently, and usually are the result of forgetting to take my medication, I can afford to stay home for a day or two and take care of myself. Though my depression is infrequently experienced to a severe degree, my entire body experiences my depression, making it less a mental phenomenon than a body phenomenon.

On the other hand, I do not always *feel* ill, although I always carry with me the *diagnosis* of mental illness. When I am experiencing depression, I certainly feel ill, but I am ill with the intensity of any other comparable short-term illness. The best analogy I have found is to think of it like the flu. I feel terrible while I have it but I know that it will soon be over. While I feel sick, I want to bury myself in bed, drink chicken soup, and sleep it all off. For me, the degree of discomfort and the duration of these two illnesses is about the same. However, when I am not feeling ill with depression, when my depression has subsided and is not with me, when my dedication is working and I feel well, I do not feel ill nor do I look or act ill. If I take care of myself, I feel good most of the time. During these times, I cannot say that I am ill. Although I am aware of my condition most of the time, the experience of illness that comes with the condition called 'depression' infrequently invades my daily life.

If my experiences with depression are not strictly mental and if I do not frequently feel ill, then the term 'mental illness' is misleading when applied to me and others like me. As I experience it, my condition is neither mental nor is it usually an illness. Rather, my condition creates one way of experiencing the world and myself within the world to which I assign another term. This term represents my interpretation of my experiences in the world. I am disabled. I do not 'have a disability', nor am I 'handicapped'. It is clear to me that I 'am disabled'.

What then, do I mean when I say, 'I am disabled'? Perhaps it helps to clarify what I am not saying. I am not saying, 'I have been disabled', or 'I will be disabled', or even 'I have a disability.' When I say 'I am disabled', I am making a distinct ontological statement of fact about my self as I understand my self at the moment of my utterance. It is a temporal claim that describes my beliefs about my self in the present and imaginable future. To say 'I am disabled' instead of 'I have a disability' is to represent my self existentially because to say 'I am' something implies a way of being, an identity, while 'I have' something implies a characteristic, or quality, of an individual that could be either separate from or related to the individual's being-ness. To question the meaning of the claim, 'I am disabled' is to raise other significant questions, particularly within the context of disabled-ness as I experience it: having a condition with intermittent symptoms that are unobservable to all but my closest confidants. It raises questions about the body, experience, and what it means 'to be' something. In the remainder of this chapter I offer some epistemological possibilities for interpreting the claim to 'be disabled', starting with a conceptual analysis of 'body' and 'experience' and then using those analyses to interpret the claim 'to be' disabled. For clarity, I approach the problem of understanding disabled-ness from my own experiences with depression, however I believe my interpretation of disabled-ness can be generalized to other disability experiences and I will examine that potential later in this chapter.

## Body

I previously established that I experience depression in my whole body and that what are commonly considered the mental aspects of depression, the mood and thought changes, are intimately connected to what is happening in the rest of my body. When I conceptualize my experiences with depression as body experiences, and when I resist medical discourses that classify me as mentally ill, I am using my body as a site of my imagination, as a means of constructing images of my self. I use the term 'self' throughout this chapter as a conceptual tool, or as a strategy for understanding the individuals to whom I am referring. So, for example, I often use the term in relation to a person (i.e. my self). When I do this I make a rhetorical decision to separate the words 'my and 'self' to indicate the uniqueness of the self and to distinguish the usage from the casual reference to one's person as in 'myself'. I am not clear that the 'self' holds a spiritual connotation, although I am open to the possibility that it might. 'Self' is not, however, synonymous with the term 'body', although I conceptualize the 'self' (whatever it is) to reside in the body or be located in the body. I am interpreting my experiences in the world through the medium of my body, viewing the body in feminist terms 'as a construct for understanding human experience' (Cooey 1994: 5) and as 'the location and artifact of human imagination' (p. 7). Within these interpretations I am the subject and object of my intrapersonal discourses. Thus, the 'interaction of site and sign in the conceptualisation of the body', or 'mapping', implies the metaphorical tension between the materiality of the world and the discourse of human relations (p. 90). As subject, I intuitively know my self and construct a view of my self as a disabled person. As object, I sit outside my self and interpret what is happening to me from the perspective of others who cannot observe my disabled-ness (because of its invisibility) and who may or may not agree with my assessment of my self. By experiencing disabled-ness in this way, as an imaginative and subjective pursuit that is influenced by my beliefs of the views others hold about me, I am actively involved in a basic human attempt to know the self.

When I understand my body this way, as something I experience and a phenomenon others perceive in subjective ways, I am allowing my body to remain somewhat ambiguous and wide open to multiple interpretations. I am echoing Rutherford's (1990) view that 'in this post-modern ... world our bodies are bereft of those spatial and temporal co-ordinates essential for historicity, for a consciousness of our own collective and personal past'.

As a creature with a liminal body, I am vulnerable to the instability of subjectivities, whether they are my own or those of others. My body, then, is constructed by my imagination and my imagination is influenced by my beliefs about the views that others hold of me. While others might form beliefs about me based on their interactions with me as well as their observations of my body, only I can experience my body while living in or with my body. My views about my body and its relationship to my self are mine alone. I am free to construct them as I wish, although my humanness forces me to be influenced by the views of others with whom I interact. If, however, I experience my body as a disabled body, regardless of what others think of me, then I am disabled. In contrast, if I do not view my body or my self as disabled, then I am not disabled, even though others may disagree. Furthermore, to view my body as a disabled body, and by extension, to experience my self as a disabled self, when I say 'I am disabled' I am making a material claim, or a claim about the real physical world as I see it and experience it. In addition, this is also an ontological claim. It is a bold statement of who I experience my self as being. As a claim about my experience of my self and my body, it is a claim that only I can make.

## Experience

In this chapter I have used the phrases 'experience my body', 'experiences in the world' and 'experience my self' without explaining my intended meaning. To do so requires an understanding of what it means to say that one has had an 'experience'. The early twentieth-century American philosopher John Dewey (1926, 1938a, 1938b) argued that there are several aspects of an event that converge to make it an experience. For Dewey, experience is not everything that happens to us. That is an interpretation of experience that is too general and has little use. Rather, experience is something to which a person gives meaning. An experience is a recognized event that is accepted as having a particular meaning with knowledge consequences. In other words, the individual having an experience gains knowledge from the experience and that knowledge influences future experiences and future knowledge. Meanings gained through experience are constructed using the tools of culture. Dewey writes that 'the things which a man experiences come to him clothed with meanings which originate in custom and tradition' (1926: 26). Furthermore, Dewey notes that experience is historical and temporal. Since experience is constructed and interpreted within a cultural, historical and temporal framework, it is contextual. It makes sense only because of the ways in which the individual having the experience interprets the world and that individual's interpretations are the result of experience within particular contexts. Experience, then, is something upon which one reflects and from which one gains knowledge of self and world.

Experience also educates. In *Experience and Education,* Dewey (1938b) argues that experience can be mis-educative or educative. The distinction between the two is in the direction of growth each promotes. Educative experiences are connected to one's past, present and future and guide the direction of growth of the individual toward future educative experiences. Mis-educative experiences are disconnected, aimless and harmful. Dewey is clear that educative experience is not always pleasant. In fact, he recognizes the struggle and pain of many human experiences. Even uncomfortable experiences can be educative, however. For Dewey, experience and knowledge of the self and the world are inextricably linked. Experiencing a thing is a requirement of knowing that thing and knowing is necessary for future experiences. This, then, is the historical context of experience.

Although clearly a scholar of his times in his implied distinctions between the mind and the body, Dewey's views on experience are provocative because for him, experience is not merely something that happens in the material, or observable, worlds. He acknowledges that experience can occur purely in the realm of thought, while he simultaneously proposes that experience is the result of a connection between thought and action. Though implying some type of duality, Dewey's suggestion of the connection between thought and action was well ahead of his philosophical times and continues to provoke debate today.

I propose that experience be interpreted, as does Dewey, as events that have meaning for the individual having experiences, where experience is understood as those events which happen and with which we construct meaning. I further propose that experience must be understood as being grounded within the body. As humans, we experience our selves and our world through the medium of our bodies. We are, of necessity, bodies, or selves within bodies. Regardless of where one stands on the nature of the self, we are encased in bodies. We move through the world in bodies. We feel through the body. We use minds that are one with, or at least intricately connected to, the body. Even those of us who cannot move our limbs or feel our toes still experience life within a body, albeit a body with sensations very different than other bodies. The body's sensations or lack of sensations, the body's movements or lack of movements, the body's functions or lack of functions, the body's emotions and thoughts are aspects of the context within which experience is had and interpreted. The human body is the medium through which we know our world and with which we experience our selves.

As a woman with depression, I have experiences with my body from which I construct meaning about my self and my world. I earlier described the physical aspects of depression in order to demonstrate that it is not strictly mental. I also described the ways in which my condition does not always feel like an illness. Depression is, however, definitely an experience. I clearly recognize body and social events that have meaning for me. They are experiences grounded in a lifetime of interacting, thinking, and reflecting. My beliefs about my disabled-ness and other aspects of my self, as well as the meanings I construct from my experiences, are uniquely my own. They are my subject-ive way of understanding and living in the world, of having a body, and of experiencing life as a human being.

In saying 'I am disabled', I am constructing my body through experience and I am interpreting my body and experience to my self and others in a cer-tain way. Disabled-ness holds particular meaning for me and 'disability' refers to experiences of my body that contribute to the meanings I construct of my self. I may use other words to represent concepts that describe other mean-ings associated with my experiences, and those, too, will have value for me, but when I use 'disabled' to describe my self, I am valuing disability and the disabled parts of me. I am saying that experiences of disability are important in the struggle to know my self and to make sense of my body's experiences. I am making a place for my self and to make sense of my body's experiences. I am making a place for my self in the world and in relation to other people.

## Being

To say 'I am disabled' is to raise the questions of being or to make claims about one's beliefs of being-ness. Another way of thinking about being or 'to be' something is to conceptualize it as identity. Heidegger (1957: 69) argues that 'the principle of identity is considered the highest principle of thought'. In making this claim, he is not suggesting that identity is merely the most inter-esting or important principle. Rather, this is a claim indicating Heidegger's primary commitment to *Being*. For Heidegger, Being is the essence of an indi-vidual's humanness, the true core of the self. The essence is related to his term 'being', which refers to any conscious person or even a particular con-scious person, but which does not refer to a specific individual's essence or individuality. A Being in Heidegger's philosophy, is fundamentally different from all other beings. All qualities of the individual are subsumed under Being. A Being is a single object, at once a sameness or a unity with the self and a difference from others that is so fundamental that the difference usu-ally goes unnoticed by the self and other beings. Being, in this framework, is one's identity. It can, however, be interpreted as a purely mental phenom-enon, as something that could theoretically exist without a body, because Being, for Heidegger, is an essence that need not be corporeal. It is not an embodiment. While Being is an ontological essence, it is the object of an epi-stemological realization. Another way to understand this is to think about the possibility that Being does not need a body to know itself, while a being might need a body to be itself.

Heidegger's account of Being, while accepting of real experience, does not depend upon the body of beings and the importance of experiences of the body and identity. First, integrating the body and body experiences into identity constructs is particularly crucial for understanding disability since disability is an experience of the body. Second, the assumption that there is an essence, which Heidegger labels as Being, is problematic from the non-essentialist perspective, or from the perspective of those of us who are uncertain about the essentialist position. Interpretively and non-essentially speaking, Being could be many things or could be nothing at all. Third, Heidegger considers what it means to be human separately from how a human knows s/he is human and how s/he understands his/her world. In effect, this disconnects ontology from epistemology. Heidegger offers a theory of identity that focuses on a *being*, an individual, but that does not connect the individual's being-ness with his/her *knowledge* of being-ness. In addition, Being can exist disembodied, though not ahistorically. In other words, although Heidegger's Being does not need a body to exist, Being does need experience, although that experience can be strictly mental.

I propose a body-centred interpretation of identity as an experience. This is a view that can accommodate the ambiguities of being a body and a self (something Heidegger does only partially) but that accounts for the necessity of experience to give meaning to body and self. From this perspective, when I say 'I am disabled', I am making a claim about my inner-most self, whatever that might be to me. I am saying that my disabled-ness is an integral aspect of who I am as a person. I am defying what others might say about me because I value what I believe about myself. I resist the outsider's view, if it disagrees with mine, and I cling to an ideology that places the view from inside disabled-ness at the center of my ideological framework.

*Being* is the active mapping out of the territory of my body, my experience, and my self. If I claim 'to be' something, then I am discursively revealing my self. I am placing my self within view of all who hear my claim. 'I am disabled', if uttered as the result of the struggle to know my self, is a claim I must make if I believe it to be true and it must be uttered regardless of the consequences. It must be written into an identity narrative I author freely, whether or not others view me as disabled. In the end, my body is my own and my experiences are mine to construct, regardless of the social powers exercised upon me. 'To be' something, disabled or female or mother, 'to be' anything, is the result of having and interpreting experiences from within my own body. Therefore, I am the most informed author of my self.

## Conclusion

In conclusion, what does this mean for the discourses of mental illness and disabled-ness? First, it provides some philosophical arguments against interpreting mental illness or disabled-ness based on appearances. Put another way, I have argued against an empirical definition of the disabled identity while I simultaneously have argued, first, for the assignation of disabled-ness by the individual experiencing the disabled identity. Second, my analysis argues against a common application of constructivism in disability studies, wherein we lament the social pressures that force individuals to be identified as disabled. Rather, I have indicated that even in the face of social control, we remain intellectually free to shape our beliefs about our experiences and our selves because that is the very meaning of experience. Finally, I have indicated that even though disabled-ness should not be based on appearances, nor should it be considered an empirical fact, it is still a body-based experience and as such, it is fundamentally grounded in the physical world, albeit a world experienced and interpreted by the individual through interaction with social others. The claim 'I am disabled' is, in essence, a statement of resistance to those who would label or construct me in the image they have created of me. This is its discursive importance. It is my construction of my being.

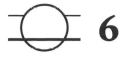 **6**

# Narrative identity and the disabled self

## Carol Thomas

### Introduction

> While Disability Studies has presented a dichotomy between the medical
> model and the social model, few have raised the issue of individual
> psychology.
>
> (Shakespeare 1996: 103)

Like many sociologists, I have tended to observe the disciplinary boundaries demarcating the various social sciences, and topics like self-identity
have been 'left well alone' (bracketed in my mind as the territory of social
psychologists, philosophers, and literary theorists). I now recognize that
these boundaries are restraining, and would like to engage with the issue of
personal identity formation – *but* with a heavy sociological slant. But how to
do it? And how to do it in the field of disability studies without falling into
individualized models of disability? This chapter is a small piece in the jigsaw.

This change in perspective is associated with my current research on disabled women's experiences of living in a disablist and exclusionary society
(Thomas 1997a, 1997b, 1998). It has become increasingly evident that as well
as drawing on (comfortingly familiar) socio-structural approaches in the
analysis of disabled women's social locations and experiences, I needed to
complement this with approaches which enabled me to make sense of the
*psycho-emotional* aspects of life which disabled women recounted to me. I
wanted to make sense of these aspects of life in terms of *disability* (as socially
understood) rather than in terms of living with *impairment* per se (that is, in
terms of a medicalized discourse of the difficult 'personal' consequences of
being ill or impaired). However, it was not only the psycho-emotional dimensions of other women's lives which were under consideration – I also needed
the conceptual tools to think about (my) self as a disabled woman. Of course,
in what follows, the latter is what really finally determines what I say about

the former: like all sociologists I inevitably construct an account which inter-prets other women's experiences according to the contours of my own intel-lectual and experiential biography (Stanley 1990; Skeggs 1995).

Self-identify is a key element in what I have termed the psycho-emotional consequences of disablism. By these I mean the 'personally or inter-subjectively felt' effects of social forces and processes which operate (not in a direct, mechanical or uni-dimensional way) in shaping the subjectivities of people with impairments. They contribute powerfully to the sense that each of us has about 'who I am' (or am prevented from being). Poststructuralists would refer to these social forces and processes as the discourses, or discur-sive practices, through which our subjectivities are produced. Rather than adopt such a perspective here, I prefer to examine disabled women's self-identities through the sociological insights in Margaret Somers's (1994) paper 'The narrative construction of identity: a relational and network approach'. Somers's analysis, though it does not address disability directly, can be applied to disability studies in a number of ways. The following extract is a useful starting point:

> scholars are postulating something much more substantive about narra-tive: namely, that social life is itself storied and that narrative is an *onto-logical condition of social life*. Their research is showing that stories guide action; that people construct identities (however multiple and changing) by locating themselves or being located within the repertoire of emplotted stories; that 'experience' is constituted through narratives; that people make sense of what has happened and is happening to them by attempting to assemble or in some way to integrate these happenings within one or more narratives; and that people are guided to act in cer-tain ways, and not others, on the basis of the projections, expectations, and memories derived from a multiple but ultimately limited repertoire of available social, public, and cultural narratives.
>
> (Somers 1994: 613–14)

Clearly, I can only scrape the surface of such application here, but for fur-ther examples, see the work of Ken Plummer (1995) on the sociology of story-telling. In this chapter I will draw on Somers's approach to consider 'narrative identity' as manifest in some of the personal accounts which dis-abled women have shared with me in the course of my research, but first it is necessary to explain how I came by these personal accounts.

## Disabled women's personal accounts of living with disability

Disabled women volunteered to tell me about aspects of their lives in response to a press release sent out in January 1996 to over 150 disability organizations (mainly national ones) listed in the *Disability Rights Handbook 1995/6*. The press release told women that I was undertaking research for a book on women and disability, that I was a disabled woman myself, and that I was looking for first-hand accounts of living with disability so that 'women's voices' could be represented in my work. It listed 15 areas of social and personal life. These items played not a prescriptive but a facilitating role, and I am certain that by naming areas such as 'sex, sexuality, sexual relationships' and 'abuse – physical, emotional, sexual', women were 'given permission' to communicate about very private or painful personal experiences that otherwise they might have kept to themselves.

Women were invited to write to me, to send a self-recorded tape, or communicate in some other way. I received written material from 49 women, self-made tapes from 5 more, and conducted 14 interviews (68 in total). The 'sample' of participating women is not statistically representative of disabled women in British society. However, ages were fairly evenly distributed through the 20s, 30s, 40s and 50s, with a few in the 60s and 70s. There was also a very wide range of physical and sensory impairments represented (my research does not extend to learning difficulty). The variable geographical location of the women was pleasing, as was their differing socio-economic, educational and familial experience. Sexual orientations differed and personal circumstances varied enormously. However, it is important to note that none of the women who communicated with me by letter or tape told me that they were Black or from a minority ethnic group (and those that I met were White), so the 'sample' might be exclusively White. I may have failed to reach and engage the interest of such women and the absence of their stories is a major omission (the press release was purposively sent to 'Black' disability organizations). Nevertheless, despite its shortcomings, the 'sample' of women who entered into dialogue with me constitutes a hugely variable yet at the same time 'ordinary' cross-section of disabled women. The material so obtained was extremely rich in form, detail and scope, providing an invaluable resource for my research. I can only refer to a fraction of it here.

**Narrative identity**

'Categorical' approaches to identity have characterized academic work on identity politics – that is, approaches which associate an individual's identity with singular (and essentialist) categories like 'race', 'sex', 'gender', 'class' (or disability); previously, sociology has been antipathetic both to 'narrative' (because of its 'discursive', 'non-explanatory' and 'non-theoretical' associations) as well as to the topics of being and identity (seen as the domain of psychologists and philosophers). In contrast to both approaches, Somers argues in favour of reframing the narrative concept in such a way that its epistemological and ontological significance is highlighted:

> These [new approaches to narrative] posit that it is through narrativity that we come to know, understand, and make sense of the world, and it is through narratives and narrativity that we constitute our social identities . . . [All] of us come to be who we are (however ephemeral, multiple,

and changing) by being located or locating ourselves (usually unconsciously) in social narratives rarely of *our own making*.

(Somers 1994: 606)

Somers identifies four dimensions of narrativity: ontological, public, conceptual and metanarratives. Three of these are particularly pertinent here,
briefly summarized as follows. *Ontological narratives* are 'the stories that
social actors use to make sense of – indeed, to act in – their lives. Ontological
narratives are used to define who we *are*, this in turn can be a precondition
for knowing what to *do*' (p. 618). Ontological narratives are produced
through the interaction of the inter-subjective with social narratives (social
narratives being both 'public narratives' and 'metanarratives') in time and
space.

*Public narratives* 'are those narratives attached to cultural and institutional
formations larger than the single individual . . . however local or grand' (pp.
618–19). In relation to disability and impairment, public narratives of particular relevance would include: the 'personal tragedy' story; medical narratives
about 'abnormality', 'deformity', 'rehabilitation' and 'adjustment'; the
'shame of the imperfect body' story (and its opposite; the body beautiful narrative); the 'it's best if you conceal imperfections' narrative; the 'dependency'
story; the 'lives not worth living' narrative, and so on.

*Metanarratives*
refers to the 'master narratives' in which we are embedded as contemporary actors in history and as social scientists. Our sociological theories
and concepts are encoded with aspects of these master narratives –
Progress, Decadence, Industrialisation, Enlightenment, etc. – even
though they usually operate at a presuppositional level of social-science
epistemology or beyond our awareness. These narratives can be the epic
dramas of our time: Capitalism vs. Communism, the Individual vs.
Society, Barbarism/Nature vs. Civility.

(p. 619)

Metanarratives of importance here are the grand narratives which
underpin the disablist public narratives listed above, involving, as they do, the
very demarcation of what it means to 'be impaired' (the social construction of
impairment), to be a 'whole' or 'less than whole' human being, and thus to be
an 'acceptable' member of the community.

## Accepting the impaired and disabled self

With Somers's conceptual framework in mind, let me now introduce a selec-
tion of extracts from the personal narratives shared with me by disabled
women. I also include a fragment of my own story (all names, except my
own, have been changed). I have selected these extracts because they are particularly telling on the issue of narrative identity and disability.

*Joan, with ME:*

I have become a stronger person mentally through ME. Learning to live
with any chronic medical condition does take a long spell of readjust-
ment. Particularly in mid life. I had a career as one of the fully skilled
'girls' within the technology industry. I lost a hell of a lot. Career, prestige and financially. Readjusting was difficult. I knew that I had a physical problem. I did five years dance training as a child. I'd been used to
using my body well. I had had an excellent speaking voice and done a
lot of movement and choral singing. Due to surgery (a thoracotomy at
the start of ME) I lost my singing voice completely. My mobility had
always been good and as a family, I, my husband and two sons had
always walked. Now a hundred yards was a long way. After three and a
half years of trying to return to a working life, and collapsing with total
exhaustion, I was frustrated. When I eventually got a diagnosis I was
firstly ecstatic that there was a name for my problem, then I tried to
ignore it. Eventually when another physically disabled person pointed
out my disabilities to me, I realized that I could no longer hide them.
Then I was so angry – why me? Having joined the ME Association, I
talked to several other people with ME and it was only after this, that I
could come to terms with it. It was at this time that I was asked to start
the local county's ME group for the ME Association.

(Letter)

Joan's story is one of changing self-identity – first the loss of the self she
was before her illness, then the reconstruction of a new 'stronger' self. We can
see this being played out through and against the public narratives of 'normality'. Before she was ill she excelled by the standards embedded in the
social narratives which constituted and sustained her ontological narrative –
a successful career, a body beautiful (movement, singing), and the features of
a 'wholesome family life'. Her difficult struggle to 'come to terms' with the
changes in her life and an altered self are clearly bound up with her long-
standing acceptance of the implicit messages in these public narratives about
'the impaired body and person': not normal, of lesser value, impaired people
as 'other'. When she became one of these 'others' her ontological narrative
was shattered and she had to reconstruct her self-identity. In this process *new*
public narratives which countered the dominant ones came into play – those
told to her by other people with ME – and she found a way to re-tell her story
to and of herself.

*Sarah, polio at 1 year of age:*

I guess I received many of the messages common to a girl brought up
between the mid-1940s to early 1960s about what a young woman
should look like and be like . . . I was always invited to friends' parties.
These were not very happy experiences. The emphasis was on appearance, dancing and the ability to attract a desirable male partner and the
playing field certainly wasn't level for me. I had no disabled friends and
few disabled acquaintances and tended to avoid 'them' like the plague. I

still have some difficulty over this. Long ago I recognized that being
close to other disabled people, especially those with similar impairments, was too like looking into a mirror. I have come a long way on this
but expect it will be a life time's work to fully accept my appearance. Of
course age adds complications and compensations to this. I know I'm
not attractive, I can dress well and look good but never to the standard I
have in mind. Part of this I think, is to do with the high priority given to
physical good looks, dressing well and the importance of sport by my
family and by the circle they mixed with when I was young. I know
many people, I mean able-bodied people, suffer agonies they tell me
when they try on new clothes to look at their perceived imperfections
in the mirror. If I hear their complaints I want to say, and sometimes
have 'You think you've got problems.' I know about inner beauty, about
beauty in the eye of the beholder, I even affirm now my own beauty.
But if you ask about my image, many disabled people feel the full negative weight of our society's notions of what is acceptable appearance
which can wound very deeply. Two years ago I attended a self-chosen,
year-long course on training the trainers in assertiveness. At one point,
two thirds of the way through the course, we were asked to draw how
we saw ourselves naked, highlighting the bits we liked and the bits we
didn't. For a long time I couldn't do it and sobbed and sobbed and
tapped a depth of emotion and pain that had been bottled up a long
time . . . Turning 50 almost exactly coincided with at last acknowledging
that disability and I were inextricably linked. I have been an equal
opportunities trainer, focusing on race/gender issues (my job description). Now I'm involved in disability equality work.

(Letter)

Sarah's ontological narrative, only recently reconstructed after many
years, is intricately bound up with public narratives and metanarratives concerning gender and disability. Her sense of (her)self as a girl and younger
woman with an impairment was constituted through the social narratives (in
time and place) of femininity, bodily normality, the valuing of sporting
prowess, and an antipathy for impaired bodies (gendered disablist discourses). She had a keen sense of 'failure' by the normality criteria in these
narratives, but was able to sustain a fragile ontological narrative, not least by
avoiding other people with impaired bodies whose presence threatened to
fracture her fragile self-identity. We can see from Sarah's account that the
(ongoing) process of relinquishing a long-held personal narrative and
replacing it with a positive one which acknowledges her impairment and
affirms her own beauty has been an emotionally painful one. Once again,
new narratives play a critical role, not least the narratives promoted in the
'trainers in assertiveness' course she attended. We are not told what these
particular narratives are but her account suggests that they emphasized
self-acceptance, and the valuing of ourselves for 'who we really are'. Sarah's

ontological narrative has recently been further rescripted through her access to the counter-narratives of disability rights.

*Karen, with MS:*
Although I am extremely embarrassed to admit it now I was reluctant to define myself as disabled, carrying as I did all of the prejudices I had somehow adopted in my able-bodied days. Coming from a liberally minded background had not enabled me to avoid these. But applying for my green form was not so difficult . . . Gradually I became a little more aware of the issues involved in disability politics. I read Alan Sutherland's book *Disabled We Stand* written in the early days of the disability movement in this country. I chanced upon mention of the local disability organization in the city where I lived and joined. I subscribed to the BCODP journal *Rights not Charity* . . . I have a great deal more to learn but in many respects my developing MS has had a very beneficial effect upon me. I am now involved in arguably the most pressing civil rights issue in this country and internationally. I am developing friendships I might never have had. If I can stop myself trying to cling on to the past and being scared of new directions I hope I can give back just a little of what I owe other disabled people past, present and future.

(Letter)

*Sally, with cerebral palsy:*
[In this job . . .] It was the first time I had had any contact with people with other disabilities and I benefited a lot by talking about my own experiences and listening to theirs. I suddenly wasn't on my own. They all seemed proud to be disabled and it was a part of them and for the first time realized that I was who I was because of my disability and that it could be a positive thing. For the first time I felt proud to be disabled in a strange sort of way . . . Now it just feels as if I've overcome it and accepted that it's part of me and I no longer have to fight it or become embarrassed by it.

(Letter)

Karen's and Sally's stories offer further confirmation that reconstructed ontological narratives are built up through accessing counter-narratives about disability and impairment – the narratives of the disabled people's movement, or just the stories told by other disabled individuals. Karen's account reminds us that self-affirming ontological narratives, once re-forged, are not fixed and static – they have to be continually worked at if they are to be sustained in the face of more dominating disablist social narratives. Sally's account reveals the power of another public narrative, or perhaps it is a metanarrative: 'one should fight heroically to overcome adversity'. She can now say, 'I no longer have to fight it', meaning that she no longer sees her impairment as a 'tragedy'.

Finally, here is a fragment of my own story.

*Carol, born without a left hand:*

I was born without a left hand, an impairment which I began to conceal at some point in my childhood (probably around 9 or 10 years of age). This childhood concealment strategy has left a long legacy: I still struggle with the 'reveal or not to reveal' dilemma, and more often than not will hide my 'hand' and 'pass' as normal. But concealment carried, and continues to carry, considerable psychological and emotional costs and has real social consequences. This hiding strategy was partly bound up with school life, but looking back I think a key influence was my association with the 'Roehampton Limb Fitting Hospital'. Once a year from a very young age I was taken by my parents to this hospital. My parents felt it was their duty to do this for my sake: to seek the advice of 'experts'. On these annual visits, my 'hand' was examined by a doctor who I remember as being very kind, and questions were asked about how I was 'managing'. As a result of these visits I was kitted out with a number of 'aides' like a strap which went around my left 'wrist' in which a fork could be inserted so that I could eat with 'two hands' like everyone else! The main 'prize' of these visits, however, was a series of artificial, or 'cosmetic' hands. These were ghastly, heavy and uncomfortable objects which I invariably relegated to the drawer soon after receipt. By the middle of my teenage years I had a gruesome collection of hands in the drawer. It was only some years later that I finally threw them away. I remember standing in front of a full-length mirror gazing at myself with the latest cosmetic hand on – how strange and unnatural it looked. Fortunately my parents never pressed me to wear these hands – leaving it up to me to make the decision. You could count the number of times I wore these on the fingers of one hand! However they did their work indirectly because the underlying message was clear. The experts were saying that my 'hand' was something to be hidden, disguised. I had to appear as 'normal' as possible. I found the easiest solution was to hide my 'hand' in a pocket, and I became very skilled at this concealment. Thereafter I always had to have clothes with a strategically placed pocket. So it was, and so it is.

As well as reflecting the gender narratives of my time, this account also tells us something about the public narrative that 'out of sight [is] out of mind'. I would suggest that this social narrative operates powerfully in relation to people who have impairments that can be, or by their very nature are, hidden, but it is a narrative of much broader significance in Western culture: conceal that which is 'bad' or shameful, make things appear to be 'normal'. In my case, doctors and others in 'caring' positions were conduits of this narrative because it was embedded in their own professional and personal identity narratives. My own ontological narrative, like those of the others discussed, has been retold through and in the new public narratives associated with the disabled people's movement. However, one of the difficulties in sustaining it, or rather in 'acting it out', is that the long history of 'hiding' my impairment has meant that it is 'second nature' to me now. There is thus a disjuncture between my sense of 'who I am' (a disabled woman) and the sense of 'who she is' held by most other people who know me. This means that much of the time I feel that I am in the 'borderlands' between the disabled and non-disabled worlds, and I suspect that this is a very common experience for people like me who have impairments which, for one reason or another, are not obvious.

## Endings

By examining the ontological and social narratives etched into these personal accounts, I do not want to give the impression that disability and impairment are the only, or necessarily the main, dimensions of relevance in our lives. As Somers (1994: 606) says, '[All] of us come to be who we are (however ephemeral, multiple, and changing) by being located or locating ourselves (usually unconsciously) in social narratives rarely of our own making.' Numerous other social narratives – all produced in particular social times and social spaces – interact to constitute the ontological narratives of those who live these times and spaces (narratives about gender, age, class, 'race', social status, place and so on). So, for example, the counter-narratives to the gender order offered by the Women's Movement have also played a key role in an earlier reconstitution of my own ontological narrative. Perhaps the key point is that without the counter-narratives of others who challenge social 'norms' we, as isolated individuals, are trapped within the story-lines of the prevailing narratives. If we do re-write our own identities then we strengthen the counter-narrative, and the dominant and oppressive social narratives begin to crumble: 'Oppressed people resist by identifying themselves as subjects, by defining their reality, shaping their new identity, naming their history, telling their story' (bell hooks, cited in Plummer 1995: 30).

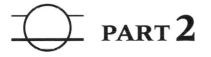 **PART 2**

# THE SOCIAL CREATION OF DISABILITY IDENTITY

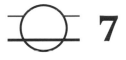 **7**

# 'Why can't you be normal for once in your life?' From a 'problem with no name' to the emergence of a new category of difference

**Judy Singer**

## The autistic spectrum

There was something odd about my family. From the first, we seemed to be marked for failure and even tragedy. All our efforts at finding friends, or making money, or having any influence in the world, seemed, bewilderingly, doomed. My parents ascribed their misery to the losses of exile to Australia, to a lack of assistance, family and community in their new 'home', and above all, to the evils of capitalism. Although I was largely convinced by the family mythology, and spent my childhood drowning in grief and loss, I still insisted that many of our problems emanated from my mother, who I was sure 'had something wrong with her'.

From the beginning, my mother confounded some expectation I had about what a human being ought to be like: how can I explain or prove the deep, innate, sense of 'wrongness' that I felt as a child, when I had no words to describe what it was about her that so violated my sense of 'rightness'? How to describe what it was like to live with someone whom everyone avoided, yet who I was never allowed to describe or ask questions about? How to write this article, without once more, opening myself up to the painful experience of having the validity of my observations scrutinized and questioned?

How can one paragraph do justice to a childhood with a parent who seemed to come from some parallel universe, similar to the one the rest of us inhabited, but tantalizingly, indefinably, different? How to honour the pain of this experience of being in the power of someone who had no sense of the needs, the separateness, the minds of others, how to describe the revulsion that welled up in me towards someone whose body language was so strangely, repellently, Other? How can anyone schooled in relativism sympathize with the frustration of having to interact with someone who seemed to have no concept of the rock-bottom, bleeding, 'obvious'?

Sure, I can describe all this, but my efforts remind me painfully of a history I just want to forget, a history of being told, 'Sorry, you're not in the textbooks, you don't exist.'

Welcome to the singular world of struggling alone with a 'problem with no name'!

Maybe I can just say, that when I first read, at the age of about 11, the words 'mental cruelty', I clung to them. Yes, it was possible that someone somewhere might have an inkling of what I'd been through. I experienced my mother as being relentlessly cruel. Not physically cruel, nothing literal-minded like that, for I knew she adored me, but 'cruel' through invasively, relentlessly, boring and stupefying the rest of us to hysterical exhaustion.

My father's response to my persistent demands that he 'do' something about it, take her to a psychiatrist, divorce her, anything, was to deny, with increasing agitation, that there was any problem. His response was, 'everybody's just different, you've got to accept people the way they are'. Yet he spent his life furiously, hopelessly, desperately exhorting my mother to 'act normal'. We had a daily mantra, that we chanted at her with monotonous regularity: 'Why can't you be normal for once in your life?'

As soon as I was old enough, I took myself to the State Library to 'look her up' in the psychiatry textbooks. Although I became an instant pre-teen expert on every kind of psychological deviance, I could find Nothing . . . 'Nothing about her case'. What could I do but abandon myself to the conclusion that everyone else around me had drawn, that my mother was just a 'bad, lazy, person who wasn't trying hard enough'? I decided she had made some wrong moral choice in her life, then got further and further out on a limb of laziness, denial, and idiotic 'fuss'.

A life full of chaos, uproar and misery made me a suitable candidate for 'therapy'. All of the therapies I went into encouraged me to think that my parents had 'chosen' their behaviour. I was desperate enough for any kind of help to cling to this idea, trying to stifle my doubts, and, when I couldn't, feeling even worse about myself: now I was a 'failure' even at therapy. My 'therapists' exhorted me to dump my mother, and abandon her to the consequences of her 'choices'. That was going to be the only way she would ever learn . . . But no matter how desperate I was to shed the burden of a bottomless importunate soul, I couldn't, for my mother had the awesome power of the *truly* helpless. Even though I simultaneously berated her for shamming . . .

I hung in a limbo between escape and responsibility, trying to hang on to the idea that I was a good person, and that one day, understanding might yet come in undreamed-of ways.

Eventually, I had a daughter of my own. By the time she was 2 years old, it was becoming obvious that my child was not 'unfolding' like the other children I observed. One day, I read an article about infantile autism. My heart froze. It seemed to be describing my daughter. Yet, my daughter was deeply loving and lived to cuddle. So surely it couldn't be autism?

I confided my fears to a friend. The hostility of her reaction taught me not to confide any new hypotheses about my daughter to anyone. Mothers, no matter how educated, were not supposed to 'compare', let alone make empirical observations about their own children. In my milieu, there was only one acceptable explanation for any kind of behaviour that deviated from the norm: an enlightened version of Terrible Mother Syndrome – 'if you come from a dysfunctional family, you inevitably pass it on to the next generation. To heal the wounds, you have to start by admitting it . . .' And I was refusing to admit anything, because I knew I was just fine as a parent. My refusal to 'confess' meant that I was to all intents and purposes, excommunicated from my circle.

Meanwhile, it was becoming increasingly clear that my daughter was developing very similar behaviours to my mother. Till then, I had thought children were blank slates to be written on by enlightened, progressive mothers like myself. Now I began to be awe struck by the reality of heredity. It became clearer that we had some kind of hereditary 'disability' in the family. But what?

At first I took refuge in the camp of 'learning disabilities' like ADD (Attention Deficit Disorder). Although my daughter never quite fitted, there was enough overlap for me to at least argue that my daughter had an organic, not a psychological, difference.

My life as a parent was a battleground for various belief systems, all of which had one thing in common: an inability to come to terms with the extent of human variability. I refused to accept any of these belief systems. I decided to stick to my truth and keep searching. And I developed a thick hide.

Meanwhile I came across Ann Shearer's *Disability, Whose Handicap?* (1981), a turning point in my understanding of disability and normality. I cried many tears of recognition over the wrongs done to the disabled, ruefully recognized my own collusion and fear of the 'disabled', realized how 'normality' was policed by the mistreatment of disabled people. I learnt much about 'internalized disability oppression' through co-counselling, and had the good fortune to find a co-counsellor with post-polio syndrome, and thus, a wealth of experience on living with physical limitations that were deemed not to exist. Thus I began to explore the effects of hidden 'disability' on my life. It took me years of sobbing out the grief, shaking with anxiety, and laughing uproariously as I recalled past humiliations, to begin to find the strength to speak against the silencing of my experience, so deeply ingrained had it become. By now, groups of women, Blacks, queers, crips, had all found their voices, their communities. It seemed that only my family was left without a group to belong to, who could speak for us and with us.

During this period, unemployment forced me back to university, and I signed on to study the sociology of disability. My readings of 'social model' theorists like Mike Oliver, Irving Zola and Jenny Morris provided me with a theoretical and historical background to the insights I was making through counselling and my own experience.

Finally, I decided not to put off any longer reading Donna Williams's (1992) *Nobody, Nowhere*, an autobiographical account of an autistic childhood, which I knew would have some important message for me. I followed this up with Oliver Sacks's (1995) account of Temple Grandin, a scientist who has become a spokesperson for autistics. I was riveted. So you didn't necessarily have to have learning disabilities or lack emotional awareness to be autistic!

This time, I knew at last who my people were, and this time I would not be put off. At the age of 9 (two years after I had figured it out myself), my daughter was 'officially' diagnosed with Asperger's syndrome, currently conceptualized as being at the 'high-functioning' end of what is increasingly being thought of as the 'autistic spectrum'. ('High-functioning' meaning 'not intellectually impaired'). I now had an entry ticket to new world of people whose struggles paralleled mine.

At the same time, I had begun to turn inside out my account of my relationship with my mother. I had not 'known' her at all. Just who had been victim and who perpetrator in our family battles became complex and finally, irrelevant. We had been but 'ignorant armies, clashing by night'.

In the breathing space I found after a lifetime of struggle, a new question arose. Was it possible that I myself had 'Asperger's syndrome', whatever that was, all along? It was beginning to look like it. Odd bits of my history which hadn't ever fitted into the race/class/gender/parents-are-to-blame discourses now began to come into sharp focus. Why had I never fitted in anywhere? I hooked into the Internet, and joined various e-mail forums some for 'autistics and cousins', some for parents and professionals. I began to see that my life's trajectory fitted in closely with that of others on the autistic spectrum. Over the past year, I have been forced, willy-nilly, to re-tell myself the story of my life through a new filter, a not unpleasant, but demanding, time-consuming imperative. In doing so I have added a neurological/biological perspective to my former sociological/psychological/spiritual orientation, and have felt both enriched and exhausted by the fullness of my vision.

The process of understanding what it means to be 'somewhere on a spectrum' is still ongoing. Throughout this article I keep finding myself using the expression 'they/we' as I try to express the ambiguities of my situation. I ask myself, by what right do I speak about or for autistics? If I am on the autistic spectrum, then so is half the world, so is every shy, awkward person who would rather pursue their special interests than the pleasures of group membership. Where is the cut-off point? I live with ambivalence about 'joining up', as I weigh the benefits of a clear identity against the potential of being stigmatized, as I once stigmatized and tried to distance myself from autistics only slightly further 'out' than I was. This 'they/we' usage reflects too a wrenching inner conflict about groups which I have not noted in fellow 'truth-seekers' as they gradually dropped off and found cosy niches in the hierarchies of various liberation and new social movements/careers/

religions: deep conflicts about 'not belonging anywhere', 'yearning to belong', 'hating the sacrifice of truth, difference, integrity that all group membership inevitably demands'. My lifelong tension between wanting to be part of the group, and needing to maintain my separateness, itself becomes evidence that I am on the spectrum.

My personal struggles in the middle of three generations of women 'on the spectrum' have been part of the birth throes of a new category of human difference coming to awareness, a new way of perceiving. But what exactly is this phenomenon, why has it constellated in this particular era, and what cultural significance does it have?

## What are Asperger's syndrome and the autistic spectrum?

As befits a disability emerging for the first time in the postmodern era, the autistic spectrum has fuzzy boundaries. Not even its name has been agreed on, appearing variously as Asperger's syndrome, High-Functioning Autism, Autistic Spectrum Disorder, Hyperlexia, Crypto-sensitivity syndrome, Face-blindness, even PDD-NOS (Pervasive Developmental Disability – Not Otherwise Specified), and probably more.

While autism is associated in the public mind with images of rocking, emotionally cut-off, intellectually impaired children and 'Rainman'-like savants, a range of people who are not intellectually impaired, and may even be intellectually outstanding, are recognizing themselves as being 'somewhere' on a continuum between 'normality' and classical autism. The DSM-IV (American Psychiatric Association Task Force on DSM-IV 1994) flags 'Asperger's syndrome' (AS) as, in summary, a qualitative impairment in social interaction marked by repetitive and stereotyped patterns of behaviour, interests and activities, leading to significant impairments in social, occupational or other important areas of functioning, in the absence of significant delay in language or cognitive development.

But for most people with AS, this definition puts the cart before the horse, looking superficially at their deficits, and ignoring the causes. To them the autistic spectrum is above all a hypersensitivity to sensory stimuli, which necessitates withdrawal from a world of overwhelming sensation. As Temple Grandin (whose pioneering autobiography *Emergence, Labelled Autistic*, about the inner world of autism, has made her a spokesperson for autistics) puts it:

A defect in the systems which process incoming sensory information causes the child to over-react to some stimuli and under-react to others. The autistic child often withdraws from her environment and the people in it to block out an onslaught of incoming stimulation.

(Grandin 1996: 9)

The people who band together under this category prefer to name their condition as AS, and themselves as autistics, and sometimes, comfortably, as 'aspies', to distinguish themselves from those they have dubbed the 'NTs' –

NeuroTypicals – or 'normies'. The preference for terms like 'autistic spectrum' and 'autistics and cousins' reflects the wide variety of people who are
beginning to identify together under the banner of what they increasingly
identify as 'neurologically different'.

For me, the key significance of the 'autistic spectrum' lies in its call for and
anticipation of a politics of neurological diversity, or neurodiversity. The
'neurologically different' represent a new addition to the familiar political
categories of class/gender/race and will augment the insights of the social
model of disability. The rise of neurodiversity takes postmodern fragmentation one step further. Just as the postmodern era sees every once too solid
belief melt into air, even our most taken-for-granted assumptions – that we
all more or less see, feel, touch, hear, smell, and sort information, in more or
less the same way (unless visibly disabled) – are being dissolved.

## Why has AS emerged as a discrete entity in this historical era?

The phenomenon that is AS sits on a busy postmodern crossroads. Key factors in its emergence have been the 'voice' claimed by women as parents, the
trickle down of 'disability rights' and 'identity politics' ideas into the mainstream, and the concomitant shifts in power relations between health 'professionals' and consumers. AS arises out of the march of science and its ever
more minute empirical observations of human difference. The successes of
science, particularly in genetics and neurology, the widespread acceptance of
drugs like Prozac, combined with the beginnings of disillusion with the
promise of psychotherapy, see a shift in the 'nature–nurture' pendulum back
towards 'nature'. Above all, the democratization of information flow which is
the Internet has promoted the emergence of new ways of self-identification
for autistics.

A prime cause in the emergence of the Autistic spectrum, which I take
from my own experience, is the increasing confidence of women in their own
judgment. Lorna Wing, who is credited with first bringing AS to wide attention, talks about how autism was widely, and often devastatingly, seen
through a Freudian lens as being caused by 'cold, detached' parenting (the
term 'refrigerator mother' figuring prominently).

> The tide began to turn in the 1960s . . . parents who were independent
> minded enough to reject the idea that they were to blame for their chil-
> dren's condition came together to form parent's associations. The first of
> these, by a small margin, was the British Society for Autistic Children,
> now known as the British National Autistic Society.
>
> (Wing 1996)

At the same time that women were claiming their voices, the prestige and
authority of medicine had peaked. In e-mail lists for autistics, at meetings of
AS support groups, whether of parents or people with AS, almost everyone
has an anecdote about consulting their GP with suspicions of having some

kind of developmental problem, to be told (in effect) 'there's nothing wrong, stop being neurotic'. Far from being intimidated, most just indignantly wrote off their GPs, and kept looking. Whereas the traditional image of 'diagnosis' is of something reluctantly sought, dreaded, resisted and imposed from outside, people with 'marginal' neurological differences, clamour at the gates, self-diagnosed, and demanding to be let in.

Earning even more scorn from autistics than the mainstream medical profession is 'psychotherapy' and its fixed developmental schemas, its assumptions about free choice, its covertly blaming discourses on building 'self-esteem'. In an age where 'self-awareness' is highly valued, people on the spectrum are spearheading neurological (as opposed to psychological) self-awareness. Possibly more than any group in society, people 'on the spectrum' have been able to finally come up with the 'stronger magic' that is needed to sweep out the priesthood of the old gods of psychological causation. By posing a more powerful explanation for 'why they are not adjusted', they are able to reject the power of psychology. A frequent theme among autistics on e-mail lists is anger at having their experiences invalidated and their time wasted by expensive psychologists and 'therapists'. To the claim that their social difficulties are caused by childhood trauma or sexual repression, they are likely to respond that the difficulty is in their 'wiring' (Blume 1997a) along with social invalidation of their different ways of perceiving.

However, this preference for neurology does not necessarily mean that the medical profession will regain its former exalted position on the pedestal. Thanks to the Internet, autistics are taking diagnosis, scientific speculation, experimentation with self-medication into their own hands. News travels fast on the net about what works and what doesn't, which practitioners are good and which are not. With this sense of empowerment, some autistics are in a position to speak with satisfaction about the medical partnerships they have been able to negotiate.

## AS, computers and the Internet

Since AS is primarily perceived as an impairment of social communication, an answer to the question of how autistics communicate is: 'Face to face, often awkwardly. But on the Internet, freed from the constraints of NT timing, NT ways of interpreting body language, free from the information overwhelm of eye contact, the energy demands of managing body language, they sound, simply, 'normal', and often, eloquent.'

On the 'InLv' e-mail forum for autistics and cousins, members regularly sing the praises of the new medium that allows them to have the communication they desire, while protecting them from the overwhelming sensory overload of human presence. One woman, in response to a thread about the ideal 'country' for autistics, had this to say: 'We've already got our own country. It's a cybercountry called InLv, and it's perfect. We can interact without getting on each other's nerves – gently, carefully.'

The imagery used by autistics to describe their thought processes is often via machine/cybernetic/computer programming analogies. For instance, Temple Grandin explains the workings of her mind thus: 'It's like if I was a computer I'd have a hundred gigabyte hard drive but very little processing. You give the person extra storage but it's at the expense of processing' (Blume 1997c).

It is interesting to speculate to what extent computers themselves were developed by people on the spectrum as meeting a communicative need of their own. The popular perception of the Internet and cyber culture is that it has been developed by 'nerds' and 'geeks'. And what are nerds?

> Nerd is a term widely used to describe the sometimes socially awkward, technologically minded, gifted people who built the digital communication structures . . . [They] have generally experienced outsiderness or worse in one form or another – socially, and often in the context of schools and work.
>
> (Katz 1997)

Whatever their own views may be on the matter, 'nerds', for my purposes, are people who fit perfectly into the definition of the autistic spectrum – difficulties with social communication, specialized interests. Perhaps it is not too fanciful to suggest that we are entering an era of co-evolution with machines that opens up a new ecological niche for people 'on the spectrum', allowing them/us to flourish and come out with pride.

I am much interested by Lennard Davis's (1995: 51) (self-styledly) 'somewhat preposterous suggestion that Europe became deaf during the eighteenth century'. Would it be any more preposterous to suggest that if the eighteenth century, the age of the ascendancy of text-based communications, turned the hearing into the culturally Deaf, then the cyber age is turning NTs into the culturally autistic? Consider how computers force us to deal with an overwhelming onslaught of pure information, minus emotional cues and feedback, how they replace the complexities of intuitive decision-making with simplified, rule-based machine logic. When these simplistic systems cannot respond fluidly enough to complex realities, even NTs can be reduced to the frustrated head-banging rage which is the old hallmark of autism. If every age has its 'disease metaphor', then is autism the metaphoric 'disease' for the era of the Internet?

While medical-model literature on autism abounds, to my knowledge only one writer has woken up to the rise of autism as a cultural phenomenon. In a stimulating paper, 'Autism and the Internet, or, It's the wiring, stupid', US writer Harvey Blume (1997a) speculates about the links between an upsurge in media representations of autism, the rise of neurology, and computers. Observing signs everywhere that we are living through a 'romance between human and machine' (p. 3) where 'artificial and organic intelligence cross-pollinate as never before' (p. 4), he goes so far as to speculate that 'Neurological man is a giant step toward – and concession to – the cyborg' (p. 6). And no group of people have claimed neurology more for their own than autistics.

However fanciful the idea of the cyborg may be, it is clear that the Internet is able to supply whatever communicative capacities high-functioning autistics lack. It has begun to do what was thought impossible, to bind autistics together into groups, and it is this which will finally enable them to claim a voice in society.

## The politics of neurodiversity, AS identity

The development of the AS identity owes much to the Deaf movement, whether consciously or through a 'trickle-down' effect. Lennard Davis shows that the deaf were not constructed as a group till the eighteenth century:

> The reason for this discursive non-existence is that, then as now, most deaf people were born to hearing families, and therefore were isolated in their deafness. Without a sense of group solidarity and without a social category of disability, they were mainly seen as isolated deviations from a norm ... Likewise, the deaf themselves could not constitute themselves as a subgroup, as might outsiders such as Jews, subalterns, even women, because they remained isolated from each other and were thus without a shared, complex language.
>
> (1995: 51–2)

And the same situation is mirrored in the experience of high-functioning autistics, whose oddness may have been noted, but been ascribed to individual moral failings, bad upbringing, etc. In an article for the *New York Times*, Harvey Blume, invited onto the InLv list to spread the word about autistics to the mainstream, envisions that 'The impact of the Internet on autistics may one day be compared in magnitude to the spread of sign language among the deaf' (1997b). With their own communication medium, autistics are beginning to see themselves not as blighted individuals, but as a different ethnicity, 'In a sense, autistics are constituting themselves as a new immigrant group online, sailing to strange neurological shores on the Internet' (1997b).

A challenge for the disability rights movement materializes: how do you include people who may need the benefits of inclusion, but cannot bear the physical and emotional presence of it? The answer from their/our point of view is that we don't want to be included, we want mutual understanding, clear boundaries, appreciation of our gifts, based on what we can do, not what we can't. Perhaps as the voices of the 'neurologically different' are heard more loudly, a more ecological view of society will emerge: one that is more relaxed about different styles of being, that will be content to let each individual find her/his own niche, based on the kinds of mutual recognition that can only arise through an ever-developing sociological, psychological, and now neurological, self-awareness.

*Note*: Quotes from members of the InLv list are reproduced with their permission.

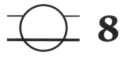 **8**

# Unless otherwise stated: discourses of labelling and identity in coming out

## John Swain and Colin Cameron

### Against the stream

This chapter is about self-labelling and identity, and we begin with an observation. In present-day Western society, the label 'disabled' differs in a crucial respect from other labels which categorize people. Whereas gender differences, for instance, have two main labels, male and female, disability is usually self-referent from only one side. In written or verbal descriptions of self (such as in the Twenty Statements Test in which people write down 20 different statements about themselves in answer to the question 'Who am I?'), many people refer to their gender; few would describe themselves as non-disabled (or able-bodied). Non-disabled is presumed unless otherwise stated. The most obvious parallel is sexual preference: heterosexuality is presumed.

It is in this context that there is a coming out process for gay men and lesbian women which has no real equivalent in gender and race categorizations. There is a similar coming out process for disabled people. It is less widely recognized because the discourse is predominantly around the labelling *of* rather than *by* disabled people – that is, self-referent labelling – except when this is understood as an acceptance of labelling by others.

The coming out process for disabled people, as for gay men and lesbian women, is a declaration of identity outside the norm, or 'against the stream'. As Corker (1996: 47) states, 'For a person who is oppressed, one of the key tasks of identity formation then involves "coming out" as different and integrating a sense of that difference into a healthy self-concept, which may, itself, be stigmatised by the majority society.' Self-declaration of identity is a coming out process when it is a declaration of belonging to a devalued group within society. Coming out has meaning against alternative processes of internalization of dominant ideologies. Within a disablist society pressures to pass as normal or to aspire to some approximation of normality, on non-disabled terms, are manifest for all disabled people.

This is our starting point for our examination of the meaning, both personally and socially, of the label and identity of 'disabled'. The chapter is in three parts, before a conclusion is drawn. We begin by outlining some personal experiences and the questions that have arisen for us in understanding their significance in terms of labels and identity. We then look at the academic literature, particularly in the field of social psychology, and review their contribution in addressing these questions. Finally we turn to the writings of disabled people and the disabled people's movement to seek some resolutions to the questions.

## Personal experiences: John Swain

I have written for a number of years in the area of disability studies. I wrote as a non-disabled person. By luck, rather than design, in the late 1970s I stepped into an arena in which ideas about disability were being debated and traditional ideas, to which I adhered, challenged. I was seconded as a lecturer to work on the rewrite of *The Handicapped Person in the Community* course at the Open University. The course team was led by Vic Finkelstein who was then a member of the Union of the Physically Impaired Against Segregation (UPIAS) and has been recognized as an influential instigator of the disabled people's movement in Britain. Vic gave me a copy of a little red book entitled *Fundamental Principles of Disability* which laid down the foundations of the social model of disability adopted by both Disabled People's International and the British Council of Disabled People. It contained the following definitions, often quoted but worth repeating:

> *Impairment*: lacking part of or all of a limb, or having a defective limb, organ or mechanism of the body; and

> *Disability*: the disadvantage or restriction of activity caused by a contemporary social organisation which takes no or little account of people who have physical impairments and thus excludes them from participation in the mainstream of social activities. Physical disability is therefore a particular form of social oppression.
>
> (UPIAS 1976)

As a non-disabled academic I became convinced that the social model provided the basis for understanding disability and the foundation for the liberation of disabled people. Over the following years I grappled with my relationship to disability as a non-disabled person, but I was increasingly to see my role as one of promoting the social model and supporting the growth of the disabled people's movement through my relatively privileged position in higher education.

Some 15 years later, in 1995, I developed insulin-dependent diabetes, and it is this experience that has raised, for me, questions of personal identity. There is no question other than that I am impaired. My impairment is a constant reality for me as I test the sugar levels in my blood daily, inject myself with insulin four times a day, and eat regular meals, watching my sugar intake. If I had been born a hundred years earlier, before the causes of diabetes were understood and insulin had been isolated, I would be dead, or at least terminally ill.

The first labelling discourse I became engaged in, then, was around impairment. It is a label ('diabetic') imposed on me, though not an identity. I joined the British Diabetic Association only to find the pages of its magazine *Balance a Lifestyle* dominated by a tragic view and the search for a cure (at the time of writing they are running a 'Campaign for a Cure') or better care. Every article and every feature reflects a medical or related (e.g. dietician) perspective, and the very title of the magazine speaks to the colonizing of a person's life. For me, coming out as disabled involved a rejection of this medical discourse of diabetes, at least as a foundation for understanding myself and my life. From the outset, I was drawn into an alternative discourse of disability.

When my diabetes was first diagnosed, the consultant made a statement along the following lines: 'You will be able to lead a normal life. Many of our diabetic patients do the Great North Run.' From supposed words of reassurance, he thus unwittingly engaged me in a disability discourse, provided me with my first personal experience of disablism, and also provided me with a good joke (if I ever aspired to normality it would not be through marathon running, whether disabled or non-disabled). In supposedly reaffirming my identity as non-disabled he drew on the dominant ideology of 'normality–abnormality', equating non-disability with normality. Since this doctor's first statement, similar views have been expressed a number of times, many along the lines that I will be able to continue as normal or that I'm no different, often with the proviso that I control myself and/or the diabetes.

Days later, a second telling response, this time purposefully stated as an ironic joke, took me further into the discourse of personal identity. On being told I had diabetes, a disabled friend laughed: 'Great. It's about time you came over to the right side.' A few months later I was invited to join Tyneside Disability Arts as a disabled member of the Board of Directors, towards a positive disabled identity, by people who were themselves disabled.

Thus my identity was claimed from both sides. To be disabled, or not to be disabled, that was the question. For me, however, the shift in disability discourse had begun a number of years before it became personal.

### Personal experiences: Colin Cameron

For those who still prefer to associate disability with personal tragedy, the major 'tragedy' in my life occurred in 1974 when, at the age of 9, I was hit by a car that was travelling at 40 mph. I spent the next 18 days in a coma, having received serious head injuries, resulting in paralysis of both hands and of my left leg. My right knee had also been badly fractured; because of the particular circumstances in which this accident took place, I did not receive surgery on my knee until about a month afterwards, by which time its repair was considerably more difficult than it would have been had it received surgery immediately. When I came out of the coma my speech was very, very slow.

Within the military hospital in which I recovered, I was assured by those who treated me that I was a 'brave little soldier' and that if I continued to 'fight' to get better, then within two years I would have 'won my battle'; nobody would be able to tell that I had been in an accident, and I would be fully well again. This, then, was the objective I set myself: two years to return to being 'normal'. At the time this sounded a reasonable proposition; I don't think I considered myself as being anything other than 'normal', I was just aware that I had been involved in a pretty damaging road accident. Two years seemed like a long time ahead but it was a date that I set myself. My aspiration was to be 'like everyone else'.

It was actually about three years later that I finally came to understand for myself that this was not a realistic option. As I rounded the corner to the school gates, having (as usual) come last in a cross-country race, I saw the rest of my class with my PE teacher cheering me home. 'Good old Colin!', 'In spite of his difficulties he still struggles on!', etc. It was at that point that I decided that I resented being defined as 'the poor boy who had the accident' and decided that, as far as I could determine it, I would be known for something else: from that point on I was rarely out of trouble. I had owned my identity as someone who was impaired, but my own way of managing this was a matter of becoming very bitter and cynical.

Within literature and other forms of cultural representation, discourses of disability and disabled people tend to be one-dimensional, dealing with stereotypes. For example, Barnes (1992) notes that the disabled person is either (a) a sad, pathetic victim; (b) a tragic but brave hero; or (c) an evil, twisted villain.

When it comes to the lived experience of impairment, things are slightly more complicated. At this stage in my own experience, I found myself being regarded simultaneously in the light of these three stereotypes (although I was not aware of these categorizations *as* stereotypes) and had to deal with them as best I could. This was the business of what Goffman (1963) has called 'the management of a spoiled identity'. As it was, I found it most comfortable to define myself and my social role in terms of category (c); perhaps I regarded categories (a) and (b) as being 'disabled' roles; whereas (c) was a role that at least I felt I had some control over. The fact that, consciously or otherwise, disabled people have to define themselves (if they have any choice in the matter at all, which is a matter of question) in such simplistic terms is, I would argue, a form of oppression.

As a teenager I experienced various problems associated with my impairment, including public ridicule, as people would laugh at the way I talked. My hands remained partially paralysed, yet I was expected to keep up in note-taking and essay-writing. As I failed to do this, so I fell behind in school work and was labelled as problematic. The reality of underachievement and exclusion from most sporting and other physical activities, within a school which placed great emphasis on competitive achievement, meant that I was unable to make my mark through officially sanctioned paths, and so instead had to fall back on the creation of devious ones. There was, too, a sense of humiliation as my peers had their identities defined in terms of everything they could do, while I felt mine was being defined in terms of what I could not do. The cumulative long-term effect of all these problems was that I believed my own bad press and developed low self-esteem and self-hatred. The perceptions of those whom I met incidentally through life, who were not aware that I had been in a road accident, were often to assume that I was just stupid, or weak, or vulnerable, and this led to various forms of abuse.

In spite of the fact that there are probably many aspects of this life with which other disabled people can identify, at this point I refused to consider myself disabled. I accepted that I was impaired, but did not regard this as constituting disability. When it was initially suggested to me that I register as disabled, I rejected this label with anger.

Having left school and pondering in what direction my future might lie, while in hospital having my left leg shortened to compensate for the loss of growth in my right, I realized that I could either remain as bitter and cynical as I was at this time, in which case I would be of no use to anybody, least of all myself; or I could take the experiences I had and the insights into life these had given, and try to use them in some way to benefit other people who might have been through similar experiences. In short, I recognized that my future would involve work with disabled people, helping disabled people, but I could not recognize myself working as a disabled person. At this stage my perception of disability was framed in terms of 'those people you see on *Blue Peter*'.

On learning about the concept of social deviancy while doing A level sociology, when I was 19, I was quite happy to identify myself as a social deviant, but not as a disabled person. Perhaps this can be regarded as a stepping stone on my route to identifying myself as disabled (as much sociological discussion of disability has been made with reference to social deviancy [Oliver 1996c]), but that time had not come. Thus, at roughly the same time as I had made a decision that I wanted to help disabled people, I was also willing to identify myself as a social deviant. With what I imagined was the noble aspiration to become a social worker, I went to Brighton Polytechnic to study for a degree in social administration. While the idea of becoming a social worker quickly lost its appeal, Brighton always seemed a particularly suitable place to practise being a social deviant.

In 1987, having finished my degree and spent a period of unemployment, I finally conceded to at least considering the idea of registering as disabled. I had been told, repeatedly, that by doing so I would make myself more attractive to employers. I went along to visit the local Disablement Resettlement

Officer (DRO), hoping to be told that I was ineligible for registration in order that, once and for all, the suggestion that I was disabled could be dropped. The DRO took one look at me and said, 'Oh yeah, you're disabled all right.' I received my green card. Strangely enough, I did not wake up the next morning feeling like a completely different person. I did not even feel depressed about it. I had not turned into a sad, pathetic victim or a tragic but brave hero. On the contrary, I felt somewhat relieved. I had recognized myself as disabled. I was offered a job the next week.

Although I now regarded myself as disabled, and was up front about the fact to people, I still regarded this as my own problem, resulting from my accident. I felt as if being disabled gave me an excuse for being the way I was. It is easy as a person with impairments to come to identify yourself as 'the problem', when all the signals and messages you receive from outside confirm this.

When, in 1992, I first came across the disabled people's movement, through the Northern Disability Arts Forum and Disability Action North East in Newcastle, I finally felt at home. I was able, for the first time, to take on the understanding that impairment is something we have, while disability is a social construction based on the exclusion of those who have impairments. I was able to recognize those stereotypes and to reject the identification of myself as a social deviant. I was able to work with disabled people as a disabled person in order to challenge and break down the social barriers by which we are marginalized, ostracized and excluded. This was what I had been waiting for and waiting to do for a long time. I had 'come out' as disabled.

## Identity discourses

In this exploration of explaining coming out as disabled, we turn next to the broad discipline of social psychology within which there are several pertinent perspectives and theories that have been applied to group membership generally, and race and gender specifically. Two theories that have generated extensive research and literature are social identity theory and social constructionism. Here we shall briefly review their possibilities and limitations in understanding a disabled identity.

Social identity theory (Tajfel 1981) differentiates between personal identity, encompassing perceived unique individual attributes of personality, likes and dislikes, particular skills and so on; and social identity, encompassing perceived characteristics of a social group. Thus coming out as disabled essentially involves a shift from identity by personal characteristics, as a non-disabled person, to identity by the characteristics of disabled people, oppressed by disabling barriers. The person's self-esteem is realized from positive, or indeed negative, individual achievements and attributes as a non-disabled person, to those of membership with the group categorized as disabled. Also the 'in-group', disabled people, becomes a more relevant source of information and social pressure.

Within the theory there are three stages of identification. The first is 'social categorization'. This is a cognitive process of recognizing the existence of two groups: disabled and non-disabled. Within the theory it is recognized that these are social categories, the product of human activity in specific historical contexts. Thus, disabled–non-disabled is not a categorization based on impairment but on the social history of disability. In the second stage, 'social identification', the process of coming out, is one of taking up an identity in your own eyes and in the eyes of others. Group membership involves a knowledge, emotional and values investment in being disabled rather than non-disabled. At the stage of 'social comparison', this investment within the group, as being disabled, becomes one of intergroup comparison. Self-esteem as a disabled person is linked to comparison with and hostility towards non-disabled people.

There are psychological aspects of coming out as a disabled person that can be addressed within the social identity theory. Each stage of categorization, identification and comparison is evident in our own experiences and the experiences of others. In particular, for many disabled people a disabled identity offers a positive self-regard in moving from a personal tragedy view to a social model of disability. Nevertheless, the theory is limited by its psychological perspective. There is no scope within the theory to account for the redefinition of disability in a coming out process, that is the political imperative of the social model. Disabled people have come out to form the disabled people's movement, to challenge existing relations and structures and the dominant ideologies that hold these in place. Thus, for example, social comparison for disabled people is not a comparison of the characteristics and attributes of one group (disabled) against another (non-disabled). It is rather an analysis of the social structures that favour some people over others.

If social identity theory offers a psychologically deterministic viewpoint for understanding the coming out of disabled people, a socially constructionist perspective can be argued to be socially deterministic. Foucault's work, for instance, analyses the large-scale creation of categories of people through the emergence of the medical and psychiatric professions. It is a perspective which provides an account (or accounts) of the creation of disability: 'Disability is a social category, which legitimates, or at the very least condones, the disempowerment of people with particular mental or physical attributes' (Gregory 1996: 360).

While this addresses the centrality of power relations and structures in disablement, it is limited in any account of the appropriation of a positive identity by individuals and collectives of disabled people.

Going 'against the stream', it seems, is difficult to explain. Academic perspectives offer only limited insights. We turn next to the understandings and explanations offered by disabled people themselves.

## Disabled identity discourse

Thomson (1997: 8) has stated that 'the term normate usefully designates the social figure through which people can represent themselves as definitive human beings'. She continues by stating that 'this neologism names the veiled subject position of cultural self, the figure outlined by the array of deviant others whose marked bodies shore up the normate's boundaries' (p. 8). In other words, in terms of a disability discourse, the social identities of those who consider themselves to be normal (or non-disabled or able-bodied) are secured only through a process which involves the systematic social exclusion and marginalization of others ('the disabled'), who are identified in terms of their deviance from an imagined ideal. The physical body is invested with political and cultural meaning and the social experience that can be expected by any individual corresponds to how closely she conforms, or can be seen to make an effort to conform, to that ideal.

The social oppression of disabled people is orchestrated through a series of techniques of exclusion and through the construction of particular discourses on disability. There are seen to have legitimacy because they have been authorized by those who 'because of the bodily configurations and cultural capital they assume, can step into a position of authority and wield the power it grants' (Thomson 1997: 8), and include: cultural stereotyping (as outlined above); identification of impairment with loss or lack of some attribute necessary to be fully human; and the assumption that treatment or cure, rehabilitation or therapy or control, pity or compensation, is always the appropriate response to impairment. Even discourses around integration serve to problematize disabled people, for there usually exists an understanding that this will involve the disabled person becoming 'more like' non-disabled people rather than a willingness to accept the disabled person for who he is.

From the viewpoint of disabled people, then, their personal and social identities have traditionally been formed within a framework from which they have been excluded. In defining parameters that state emphatically what disabled people are *not* (i.e. 'normal'), the dominant cultural discourses determine that disabled people's self-reference is measured against this. Because disability, when identified as a personal attribute, is regarded as an undesirable quality, this has led many disabled people to reject disability as a social identity for themselves and to become tangled up in various forms of self-oppression.

Three particular responses or personal strategies commonly associated with self-oppression are self-punishment, denial and passing. In Shakespeare *et al.* (1996: 54), one disabled contributor stated: 'There are a lot of things about me to do with my identity as a disabled person, not coming to terms, not coming to accept who I am . . . I was an alcoholic at eighteen, and I was addicted to gambling, I think this was all part of the punishment process, I hated myself, I couldn't stand myself, I thought I was the ugliest thing around.' Another said: 'I was in denial about being disabled most of the time, and if I saw anyone who was disabled I didn't want to talk to them, and if I did talk to them it was as if I was able-bodied talking to them, doing the old patronising bit' (p. 51). Shakespeare *et al.* argue that 'people with hidden impairments are sometimes less likely to "come out" as disabled, and move to a positive acceptance of difference and a political identity, because it is easier to maintain a "normal" identity' (p. 55). By passing as non-disabled, by minimizing the significance of their impairments within their own personal and social lives (perhaps by doing the Great North Run), people with hidden impairments often make an effort to avoid the perceived stigma attached to a disabled identity.

These responses and coping strategies are responses by disabled people to the experience of living with impairments within a world in which the dominant disability discourse is an individualizing one. Within such a context, each of these responses is valid. Each represents a way of managing identity when identification as disabled is necessarily to be devalued or to be perceived as in-valid.

The separation of disabled people into impairment-specific categories has also served to reinforce the impact of the individualizing discourse, creating a situation in which people have identified themselves as more or less disabled. The less disabled an identity that someone has of herself, the more she has been able to aspire towards 'normalcy' and the less bound she has felt herself to associate herself in her own mind with other disabled people.

The emergence of a discourse on disability around the social model and the corresponding emergence of a self-organized disabled people's movement, however, has provided disabled people with alternative frames of reference within which to build their own identities. Once the separation of disability from impairment has been established by disabled people, the process of coming out as disabled is relatively unproblematic. Another contributor to Shakespeare *et al.* stated, 'I think you can only come out when you first come into contact with an understanding that . . . you are not the problem, it's society' (1996: 57).

Coming out, then, for disabled people, is a process of redefinition of one's personal identity through rejecting the tyranny of the *normate*, positive recognition of impairment and embracing disability as a valid social identity. Having come out, the disabled person no longer regards disability as a reason for self-disgust, or as something to be denied or hidden, but rather as an imposed oppressive social category to be challenged and broken down. The forms this challenge takes are varied. They include direct political action and campaigning for equal opportunities to access education, employment, transport, housing, leisure facilities and control over personal lives; research on disability issues controlled by disabled people; and the creation of alternative cultural representations of disability through the practice of Disability Arts.

Perhaps the most significant consequence of coming out, apart from the positive impact the process has for the personal identities of disabled people themselves, is that, in the act of coming out we are changing the very meaning of disability.

## Otherwise stated

In the whole arena of disability, labelling and identity, there are many discourses – a babble of voices. Coming out as disabled can be understood as a shift or change of discourses at different levels. To say 'I am disabled' is essentially a personal statement of self-categorization, labelling and identity. Within this statement lie two changes of discourse: one is from impairment to disability (from 'I am impaired' to 'I am disabled'); and the second is from being non-disabled to being disabled. The first shift is from a medical discourse of diagnosis of impairment to a social discourse of the disabling barriers facing people with impairments. The second shift is from the dominant discourse of the abnormality and dependency of disability, to the celebration of difference and a pride in a disabled identity. In both these changes of discourse, the personal becomes political, and coming out becomes a political, collective commitment as well as a change in personal identity. As a collective process, coming out turns into collective action of protest and campaign against socially disabling barriers. As exemplified particularly by the growth of the Disability Arts Movement, a change of personal identity can become a collective celebration of and pride in being disabled.

We shall conclude by suggesting some complexities in this diverse process of coming out as disabled. First, our personal experiences have illustrated a diversity of shifts in coming out. For Colin Cameron the personal became political, but for John Swain the political became personal. From both our viewpoints, in writing this chapter we are 'otherwise stated', engaging in the positive declaration of being disabled. Second, as we have attempted to illustrate, the discourses of impairment and disability, though related, are essentially distinct. It is possible to be impaired but not disabled (e.g. short-sighted). It can also be possible to be disabled without being impaired, as in the case of many people who have been labelled as having mild learning difficulties. Third, the process of coming out, being both political and personal, varies in terms of contexts and time. Coming out at the personal level, in particular, can take years. Fourth, it is possible to be disabled, that is face disabling barriers, and not come out as disabled. If this was not so then there would be no coming out process. Furthermore, coming out, in our analysis, involves a political commitment. Acceptance of a medical model of disability and being categorized by others as being disabled does not constitute coming out as disabled. Finally, political commitment to the social model of disability and the disabled people's movement is not necessarily confined to disabled people. It is possible to be non-disabled and politically committed to disabled people.

The shift of disability discourse is the essence of our analysis. It is the context for and is given meaning by coming out as disabled. Coming out does not eliminate discrimination and oppression. It shifts the discourse from struggle against self to struggle against the disabling society. To be 'otherwise stated' is to be personally and politically committed.

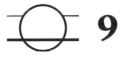 **9**

# Carving out a space to act: acquired impairment and contested identity

**Anthony Hogan**

## Introduction

Communication based on hearing and speech is part of taken-for-granted rules for daily practice. The nature of these practices structures social participation and access to culture. If language structures practice, then a subjectivity centred on deafness, on the absence of the prescribed mode of interaction, means that an individual is unable to participate in a manner expected within the social. Spoken and written language shape the core of everyday interactions to which most are accustomed. Of course, the rules of interaction governed by communication go far beyond syntax; within communication are the prescribed rules for the everyday. Acceptance, humour, anger, rejection: these are all communicated by sounds, through intonation, speed, emphasis and silence. Language constitutes people as very specific types of actors. The governance of deafness is about shaping behaviour so that the core rules and values of hearing culture, and the systems, technologies and networks that sustain it, can be secured and upheld in very specific ways.

Deafened people share a number of common experiences. Generally speaking they are born with hearing, acquire speech and develop an identity as an able-bodied person. Acquired profound hearing loss disrupts daily practice for deafened individuals and those with whom they interact in a way which projects the deafened person into a marginal social position. The extent of this marginality depends on the extent to which the individual retains usable hearing and speech skills. However, disruption is not just about communication; it is about deeply held values concerning the social position of people with disabilities where disability is perceived as a personal deficit and a moral failing. This way of understanding disability emerged during the nineteenth century and was shaped by four issues of the day. First, the nine-teenth century was a time of social upheaval. Community leaders were fearful of social uprisings by marginal groups such as people who may have been poor, homeless, criminal, disabled or homosexual. Collectively these groups were perceived to constitute a 'menace' to the security of the community (Weeks 1989; Hogan 1995). Second, a belief in moral individualism and the ethic of economic self-sufficiency began to emerge. These ideas promoted the notion that individuals were economically and socially responsible for their own subsistence and that community resources were better directed to promote the economy than to sustain welfare programmes (Fusfeld 1994). Third was the emergence of the bio-mechanical model of the body, which promoted notions that parts of the body that did not work could be repaired or replaced (Weir 1990). Finally, the latter part of the century saw the emergence of the eugenics movement (Pfeiffer 1994). Part of this movement's concern began with attempts to prevent people with disabilities from having children and culminated in the Holocaust, where many people with disabilities were executed in concentration camps. These four issues have served to shape the moral economy (Dean 1992) governing the practice of disability; a fact highlighted in recent debates concerning chronic illness, disability and euthanasia.

Acquired disability signals a massive change in a person's social position and constitutes a personal crisis for the individual. Identity as a social phenomenon becomes apparent as individuals are perceived by themselves and others as different: an experience of difference that goes beyond Goffman's notions of stigma (1963; for a critique on stigma see Finkelstein 1980). The lived experience of being deaf contests the notion that the world is hearing, a notion which follows the idea that because hearing and speech have traditionally dominated modes of communication, deaf people should also hear and speak. The experience of deaf people. in whatever form, contests ableism (a world based on values that suit able-bodied people) just as feminism contests patriarchical dominance. Ableism is therefore a political issue for disabled people (see, for example, Davis 1995: 172). However, the process by which this happens may differ for different groups of deaf people. For example, people born into families of Deaf people join a community where the right to be Deaf is validated and supported (this community, which is widely held to constitute a cultural and linguistic minority, is commonly referred to using an uppercase 'D'). People born deaf into hearing families face similar challenges to those of deafened adults. However, in their case, decisions about culture and identity are often made for them by others; a decision that many may seek to reverse in adult life (for a deeper discussion of the distinction between *deaf* and *Deaf*, see Padden and Humphries 1988).

Endeavours to create deafened people as people who use solely hearing and speech (rather than a diverse range of communication systems and technologies) – usually referred to as Oralism or the Oralist Clinic – began in earnest in the late nineteenth century (see Winefield 1987). However, deafened people find themselves acting within a new context based upon old frameworks for meaningful practice. They enter a world turned upside down by actors, embodied and institutional, who set out to (re)shape the nature, meaning and trajectory of the experience at hand. As deafened people struggle with questions of 'before and after', they do so within the context of their own historicity: 'identity stems from agency, and presupposes a continuity of practices with respect to historical conditions of existence' (Warren 1988: 199).

Acting in this context is about reconciling changes in the lived experience of social relations within available conceptual frameworks, which are managed within a context of being acted upon as well as acting, while trying to reestablish some direction in life – a direction that reflects some notion of normality.

In *Technologies of the Self* Foucault (1988) provides a framework for understanding the governance of individuals. This process includes technologies of sign systems, which permit us to use signs, meanings, symbols, or signification (p. 18). Such meaning systems are rarely homogeneous, being made up of competing and complementary value systems – hence the notion of moral economy. As individuals are affected by fluctuations in financial markets, so too are they affected by changing social values and their consequent moral implications for the self. In this chapter I demonstrate that learning to live with acquired deafness is a work of personal reformation shaped, in the Foucaultian sense, by competing systems of meaning, social production and power. Within the seemingly innocent walls of hearing rehabilitation clinics, an intense power struggle takes place. At these clinics, power is exercised as a result of the synergistic efforts of various agencies (government, insurers, technology manufacturers, professional groups of doctors and therapists, self-help groups). The mind of the deafened person, and in turn their body, are the site upon which this power is exercised. I examine how deafened people engage such technological processes as they seek to renegotiate an identity as a deafened person where their legitimacy to do so may be contested and where decisions may be made without access to the full range of choices available. To achieve this end, the experiences of three people, Carol, Sandra and Jan, are described and their process of engagement from three view points is considered – that of seeking to retain an identity as a hearing person and those of creating a dual identity, with or without the use of various technologies.

## Carol, Sandra and Jan – carving out a place to act

Acquired hearing loss sets up a paradoxical process: one is different yet one stays the same. Communication is now different but the rules for social engagement remain unchanged. Practices associated with the notion of stigma management can be taken on by the deafened individual because the ableist discourse holds that the inability to communicate in various settings is a sign of personal failure. Not of course the sign of complete failure; ableist discourse holds that complete failure is evidenced in those who use sign language. The discourse reminds deafened people that they are right to be embarrassed by their inability to converse in a fluent manner, but while they remain above the 'feral' pit of signing, they can retain some sense of dignity. A silence overshadows the experience of disability when it is construed within notions of stigma and shame. This silence skips over the difficulty of surviving a marginalizing process. It is a silence deafened people have to endure and from which they seek to escape. To stay here means to engage in social encounters in a manner deemed unacceptable, to linger continually on the borders of marginalization. This notion of being in a borderland encapsulates the paradoxical position of being both same and different (Jagose 1993). Physiologically the deafened person is different, but this is a tiny physical difference given the size of the cochlea, if not a tiny social difference overall.

*Carol*

Carol became deafened in stages, commencing with a childhood illness and culminating in a final loss in early adulthood. At 18 she acquired her first hearing aid. Carol describes her childhood as shy and socially isolated, but as though she had chosen this path:

> I was the book worm. So I sort of shied away from people, all that sort of thing.

The onset of hearing loss is often slow and progressive. This transitional process 'locks' the individual into a trajectory that is not interrupted by the onset of total deafness. Rather, the direction of the trajectory is intensified. Following the complete loss of hearing, one must work even harder to remake the self as a hearing person. It is here that the classical interpretation of Parson's (1951) 'sick role' is gathered into the morality surrounding acquired profound hearing loss. A moral obligation falls on the deafened person to participate in prescribed rituals and disciplines in order to remake themselves as hearing people. Until they are remade, they cannot disengage. The reality, of course, is that the most profoundly deafened people never regain the ease of communication they once knew and, in consequence, they are never freed from the bondage of the clinic. Nor are they considered normal, no matter how much they transform themselves. As such, an element of dehumanization remains.

Carol was ashamed of her deafened body to the point that she no longer wished to be seen by people. Deafness turned an adult experience of interaction into an experience of childhood – to be seen and not heard. Warren (1988: 148) aptly remarks that 'communication requires intelligibility and intelligence requires rule-following'. By inference, a deafened person becomes stupid because they are regarded as not having sufficient basic intelligence to participate properly in daily interactions. Carol's experience of self had been developed in the light of problematic social encounters, in the knowledge of the demands of communication environments – those already known and those anticipated in the future. Her sense of self was 'not just divided between the remembered and the forgotten, the future and the past, but between the self and the other' (Diprose 1993: 9). Carol was very much aware of this dual process. Reeling from marginalizing encounters, she remarked:

> I was becoming very much an introvert . . . I was isolating myself from people. I didn't want to go places because I knew I couldn't talk to them and so forth.

Carol avoids the detail of such encounters – the 'and so forth'. The 'and so forth' encapsulates the marginalizing process, often described using Goffman's (1963) notion of stigma and spoiled identity. The concept of stigma suggests that when a person is confronted with the threat of marginalization, they may experience a sense of shame, guilt or anxiety because they recognize that they lack something or possess something considered by others to be undesirable. The stigma response, as it were, is thought to resolve awkward moments in otherwise 'normal' interactions. Giddens (1991: 66) says that 'shame often focuses on that "visible" [i.e. identifiable] aspect of self, the body'. Historically, deafness may have been socially visualized by people wearing identifiers such as hearing aids or cochlear implant speech processors. Modern hearing aids and 'discreetly' worn cochlear implant speech processors create a setting in which such identifiers may go undetected. Deafness is most commonly visualized when spoken social interaction breaks down and in so doing threatens to disclose the gap (and all moral imperatives associated with it) believed to be embodied within the deafened individual.

Carol subsequently met other people who were in a similar situation. This group had developed skills and communication tactics generally found to be acceptable to hearing people, which supposedly meant that they could 'pass' as hearing people. Carol's feelings about herself changed as did her social activities and networks:

> You didn't have to be embarrassed about having the hearing aid sticking [out of] your ear like this body aid, like this big ear piece here or cords showing and all that sort of thing.

Carol translated the communication ideas she learnt across various aspects of her life. At work, she set up mirrors so that when she could not look directly at clients she could still see their faces in the mirror and lip-read. For her, it became a challenge to 'pass' in the hearing world on their terms. Confronted with the slide into personal dissolution, Carol set off on a trajectory that was supported by an ideological framework and social process. Carol regarded herself as more fortunate than most – the little residual hearing she retained greatly aided her ability to lip-read and therefore pass as a hearing person. Thus by behaving in a manner acceptable to the hearing world, Carol was able to gain some control over an otherwise dehumanizing process. Passing offered a limited form of liberation – that one had overcome one's disability. Self-governance was also achieved because this deafened person subjected herself to personal admonishment, adopted particular behaviours and pursued legitimated associations.

Giddens (1991: 56) points out that the essential criterion for agency is competence: 'routine control of the body is integral to the very nature both of agency and of being accepted by others as competent'. He also suggests that the opposite of shame and its associated fear is self-esteem and 'confidence in the integrity and value of the narrative of self-identity' (p. 56) – something referred to in the Deaf Community as Deaf Pride. Giddens and Goffman hold that the very promise or threat of a social encounter poses a crisis of individual identity because the person is confronted with a struggle between cultural pride and personalized shame. Identity then is a social phenomenon, a product of social engagement. Becoming deafened disrupts the narrative of personal identity. Deafened people cannot control the interactive processes in the same way as hearing people because hearing people's rules for communication are privileged over those of deafened people and because deafened people lack the necessary social organization and power to contest this relationship. Feelings of guilt and shame related to the experience of having this disability reflect the internalization of a social problem as a personal ill (Mills 1970). They reflect an unresolved dissonance within the individual because daily living cannot be reconciled with the meanings and expected behaviours legitimated by the ableist discourse.

The practical and symbolic techniques of personal understanding and formation promoted by the traditional hearing clinic sustain deafened people within problematic social relations. The privileged nature of hearing culture is not brought into question. By inference, the source of this problematic is located within the deafened person and their attention is focused on developing coping strategies to fit in with the rest of the hearing world. However, not every deafened person follows this path. In fact, it is possible for deafened people to pursue alternative communication pathways and to validate their identity as deafened people, as the narratives of Sandra and Jan show.

*Sandra*

> But I would not call myself deaf or fully hearing, mind – somewhere in
> between the two which gets a little bit awkward. It's like sitting on a
> picket fence and it gets very uncomfortable.

Sandra was in upper primary school when her hearing started to deteriorate. Sandra quickly discovered the personal price of non-conformity with these rules and her world was in chaos. She could neither understand what was happening, nor do anything about it. It created an anger within her which she carries to this day – 40 years later. The diagnosis of deafness did little to enhance Sandra's social position within the school environment. Lumbered with a large body aid, which amplified everything in the room, she

was supposed to be able to cope in school just like anyone else; reading the
teacher's lips as the teacher wrote on the blackboard! Sandra's punishment
for being deafened continued into adulthood. No one employed her. No one
was prepared to accommodate her communication needs in a workplace
which relied little on telephone work. Luck briefly changed and Sandra was
employed in a government department as a clerical worker. The position
came about as a result of a programme of affirmative action targeting disabled people. But circles of oppression surrounded Sandra, as a deafened
person and as a woman. Being deaf, Sandra was not allowed to join the workplace superannuation fund nor would her insurance company cover her for
driving a car. Sandra held her job for five years before being forced to resign
because she got married – married women were not allowed to work in the
public service in Australia until 1968. If school had not already strongly suggested to her that there was something very negative about being deaf, adult
life confirmed the reality.

As her adult life progressed, Sandra's hearing sensitivity fluctuated – sometimes for the better, other times not. Unfortunately, the management of a
fluctuating loss is not simply achieved by adjusting the volume of a hearing
aid. Sandra's loss fluctuated by frequency as well as in intensity. Sandra had
learnt to integrate visual stimuli with the little auditory input she had left,
and this had been enough to enable her to communicate. When her losses
fluctuated, so did her communication skills, until such time that she was able
to recalibrate her ears, eyes and brain:

> But then I had the shocking confusion – a doorbell. Before I used to be
> able to hear through the hearing aid – it dings! Now I hear a bit of a
> 'thawong' – and I stand there and think – what's that? What's that? My
> mind couldn't connect that sound up. It was a totally different sound.
> There were other bits and pieces. Then I found I couldn't lip-read. I
> would look at the person, but I couldn't lip-read them. Nothing would
> go in. I have since read of a woman in America who had a stroke and
> lost her sound suddenly overnight too. Same thing happened . . . her
> ability to lip-read also left her.

Fluctuation resulted in additional consequences. Sandra's capacity to communicate would also fluctuate, and this meant that people would not know
how to cope with her when her skills changed. Life took on a new level of
chaos. Stress was everywhere. With her children, her husband and friends,
confusion reigned. The loss of hearing not only constituted a loss of the self,
but also a loss of intimacy with those near to her. The resulting chaos and
incoherency was exacerbated by a medical profession that could only moni-
tor the process. They could neither predict nor control the changes.

Despite the explosive, stress-filled unpredictability of home life, Sandra
worked to maintain a 'normal' hearing family life. Sandra readily admits that
it would have been easier for her to sign and to live as a Deaf person. For
Sandra, the incoherency of 'being oral' (as she calls it) when you are deaf
does not work with little children. They cannot comprehend that one can talk

but not hear. There have never been nor still are services that help families to make the types of changes required by the onset of profound hearing loss. In Sandra's mind, this has amounted to a prejudice against a Deaf way of life. While Sandra persevered with hearing culture at home, she gradually discovered that there were other ways of being deaf. Brought up within a hearing family, deafened at a young age, engaged in medicalized processes for many years and married in a hearing family, Sandra developed strong attachments with hearing culture. However, her constant engagement with marginalizing processes set her off on multiple pathways. Reflecting on the process she remarked:

> the isolation caused my mind to take that bearing towards the Deaf mind.

What does Sandra mean by a 'Deaf mind' when her background is so steeped in hearing culture? Sandra collapsed 40 years of change into a few sentences. It is important to unpack this absence, because it is so informative. Sandra complained that there were no signposts to tell the deafened person how to cope, how to manage others, how to change others, or to tell others that they should change. For Sandra, there was not much use in talking to a hearing service provider about being Deaf – what did they know about the everyday encounters faced by deafened people within a world hostile to the overall experience of disability? For Sandra, the adjustment process was one of constant adaptation to an unstable environment, in which one needed a lot of support. Looking forward, Sandra holds that such support is still required by deafened people:

> They also need to be able to come in frequently and sit down and talk about the problems that happen with it – the hearing aid, for example – whether they [are] finding it makes their head feel it's splitting apart.

But she goes further: future services must provide an empathic connection between the provider and service user, a connection that can only come from a meeting of minds, a unity born of common experience and understanding. For example, only a Deaf person can teach another how to listen to music through feeling the vibrations! Peer support provides a forum in which the problems of hearing culture can be worked through, strategies developed, problems resolved. It is not simply a matter of counselling, but of interpersonal understanding about the overall change process the deafened person has engaged in and the mutual acceptance arising from a common road travelled. As Starr (1991: 29) remarks:

> [W]e are the ones who have done the invisible work of creating a unity of action in the face of a multiplicity of selves ... This experience is about multi-vocality or heterogeneity, but not only that. We are at once heterogeneous, split apart, multiple ... we have experience of a self unified only through action, work and the patchwork of collective biography.

Sandra has arrived at the point of having developed a Deaf mind over a long period of time. Even then, she points out that she lives in multiple worlds. Her family connections keep her firmly in the hearing world. Yet Sandra is far from being a 'pretend deaf person'. She is multi-modal: she signs, speaks and lip-reads. At home she uses a range of technologies including a telephone typewriter (TTY or minicom), and various visual alerts (e.g. flashing lights to know someone is at the door). But Sandra restates constantly the need for peer support and skills-building services for deafened people and their families. If they had been available, her life would have been a lot less stressful, and her transition to a world of multiple identity would have occurred a lot earlier and certainly more smoothly. For Starr (1991), the legitimacy of the multiple self is reclaimed by validating the hidden work undertaken to remake the self as a deafened person, by defying the construct of able-bodiment and through recognizing the benefits, the personal power and the marginality arising from living in multiple worlds. As Sandra demonstrates, the experience of the multiple self is real, it can be achieved.

The Oralist project seeks to deter deafened people from developing this multiple sense of identity, this capacity to exercise personal power; it presents it as a chasm, an abyss to be avoided:

> The big problem with the hearing person [who] goes deaf is they have been brought up with the idea that the Deaf are weird and they're frightened of moving over there. Frightened of going out on their own, frightened of having their own foundations torn up. There is still a need to bridge that gap – and it is important to still operate in the hearing world – but you are under stress . . . You've got to battle to bridge that gap yourself – so there's a real need for the deaf, the hearing people to try to move towards the deaf world, for their own good. The more they can relax, the better they cope, plus you find yourself as a person of some worth.
>
> (Sandra)

Sandra recognizes the experience of deficit endured by deafened persons who identify themselves with the hearing world. She acknowledges that the gap is fearful because it identifies an abyss into which one is jettisoned alone. And it appears that while in there, one is destined to remain alone. But as Sandra slowly learnt, one is not alone. Sandra stumbled her way through the process of being deafened, endured the battle and found places where her difference was accepted and the sense of deficit to some extent was extinguished.

At the same time, Sandra worked to maintain her connectedness with the hearing world, particularly with her children, for whom she has endured most. Sandra has found a way to achieve a sameness that does not completely disrupt her attachments with the hearing world. The sense of deficit created by the biomechanical model of the body is extinguished by engaging in a process of constantly reworking relations that produce sameness, where sameness is understood as a sense of coherency, as an experience of the continuity of self and a connectedness with others:

'Sameness' is a quality of our relation to the world, our assimilation of it, our interaction with it, and our appropriation of it. 'Sameness' is a cognitive stance that we take toward existence, a stance that is replicated and reinforced through its functioning in willing. In this case, identity is never closed or exclusive; it is never metaphysically guaranteed because it constantly must be constructed and reconstructed.

(Warren 1988: 201)

Sameness is achieved because life goes on. Sameness is produced by constant change. The issue of sameness is about finding a way to get on with things, of building new networks of people and re-establishing old ones, even if one's overall life experience has been marginalized. Sandra's life history demonstrates that the system of governance generally imposed upon and accepted by deafened adults is not all-encompassing. Sandra has carved out a place for herself in differing worlds. It is a compromise, the least worst outcome that enabled her to identify with Deaf people, and to maintain contact with her family. Sandra also considered a cochlear implant but rejected it because the benefits of implantation did not outweigh what it involved. She would still have to lip-read and could not use the telephone except in limited circumstances. She would still be too deaf to be a hearing person and she now found enjoyment and acceptance living as a deafened person. Most deafened people do not appear to arrive at this point, either prior to or after their involvement with the Oral Clinic.

### Jan

Jan suddenly acquired hearing loss when she was in her early teens. Fitted with high-powered hearing aids and placed within a mainstream school, Jan's experience of surviving school followed Sandra's. After completing initial post-school training, Jan held down a number of jobs before being laid off at age 21, as a result of a common occupational health injury. It was about this time that Jan joined a support group for young deafened adults and a process of transition began. She became quite active within the group and took on organizational responsibilities. But Jan did not find the group satisfying, particularly because it met infrequently, leaving her with many unfilled hours each day. Bored with her life, she left and became involved with a voluntary service organizing services for Deaf people. Here, Jan was surrounded by signing Deaf people and she began to sign herself. During this time, Jan also got a cochlear implant and became involved in providing peer support for other cochlear implantees.

Like Sandra, Jan stresses the importance of having access to people who have 'walked the talk', that is, people who have been through the process of having gone deaf and of having to select new ways to communicate and sustain a positive life. Jan identifies other people who, unlike herself, have not moved over or who are very much caught in a borderland between Deaf and hearing worlds, who continue to judge themselves against an ableist model of what being a hearing person might mean and in doing so, finding themselves lacking – in debt as it were (Diprose 1993) to hearing society.

Jan's experience of deafness and family life reveals a process of emotional and social divestment that is coupled with an emergent Deaf identity. For Jan, her deafness, the most structuring aspect of her life, could not be discussed at home:

> [My deafness] was just never talked about. I don't really know what they feel because we've [never] sat down and talked about it. And it was funny. I made the observation, I turned 26 last year and I realized that at that stage that I had spent exactly half of my life hearing and half of my life deaf! No that sounds weird doesn't it! Yeah. And I told that to my mum ... and you should have seen her she was so ... how do you put it, shocked. She'd never thought about it. But she immediately switched herself off. So I don't think I've ever really thought about it.

Starr (1991) suggests that the experience of multiple selves serves as a critical point of analysis for understanding the taken-for-grantedness of everyday interactions and the so-called stability of social practices which are in fact quite unstable for many people. For deafened people, it is the very taken-for-granted experience of communicating verbally on a daily basis that creates an experience of marginality. For deafened people the hearing world is distinctly not ordered. Rather, it is a source of chaos and trouble (Starr 1991: 42). Jan was marginalized at family social gatherings, finding herself left in the kitchen looking after the catering. During school life, male students did not want to be associated with her either. Her partner to the school formal dance stood her up. Aware of the communication problems she encounters, Jan aptly remarks:

> Well, like most people with a hearing problem, you stick me in a group of people, hearing people. You can't keep up with the conversation. Umm, I sometimes get upset about my ... I suppose I listen to my parents too much, sometimes. But I suppose I get upset about my inability to be able to keep up with their conversation in a group. But with my friends, no problems at all because they know, well they know me. So it seems funny that my friends know me better than my parents do, yeah.

Who are Jan's friends? Well, most of them are Deaf and deafened people who are involved in the various movements she has joined. Jan's emotional stake in home is still high – these people are family. But like Sandra, Jan draws emotional satisfaction from her new network, while retaining an attachment to the old. Jan describes this network as a solid group of people on whom she can rely for support and understanding. For Jan it is also a two-way street, for she clearly gives a lot of support to people as well:

> The benefit of being with deaf people is that in some ways we've still got the same problems with hearing people. I mean if we're speaking with someone and you can't understand something and you ask them to

repeat it, you're not treated as if you're stupid or that you have no IQ or you have absolutely nothing between your ears except cotton wool, which often happens with hearing people. Hearing people just cannot seem to understand that it is a communication problem. The fact that I have a full brain of brain cells and they are all working is not relevant. It's simply because it could be anything. Someone could have walked between us or all of a sudden some background noise could have started up or they went like this and covered their mouth or it could be anything, they could have turned away or they could have said a word I may not have caught. All of that does not occur to hearing people at all. With deaf people, you are generally accepted for what you are. And I've got a strong network of deaf people that I can count on for support. Um, have friends with [and] go out and rage. Um, or simply just talk to. Some are implantees. Some are mildly hearing impaired. Some are full deaf, some are in between. It's just a mixed bag.

Jan describes herself as a person with two passports, one into the hearing world and one into the deaf world. Her communication skills enable her to move between the two. Each world brings with it benefits and hassles:

I could not spend all of my time in either world. I just could not pick one or the other. So when I get sick of hearing people I go and mix with deaf people and when I've had enough of deaf people, I go and mix with hearing people. So I consider myself lucky and privileged that I am accepted in both.

## Concluding remarks

Sandra and Jan's life histories problematize the classical notions of Deaf and hearing worlds. Although their lives appear to be quite different, Sandra and Jan's worlds are both Deaf and hearing, never being entirely one or the other. They have moved beyond the commonsense world of Oralism to take up aspects of Deaf culture while retaining distinctive Oral traits such as lip-reading, the cochlear implant, flashing lights, hearing dogs, hearing and speech. The activity of moving between worlds is significant. Moving over is an ongoing, active process where individuals construct themselves in response to the communication environments encountered. As Warren (1988) points out, agency enables the individual to differentiate between practices which benefit as distinct from those which disadvantage. Thus the process of equipping oneself for communication is about fabricating one's identity; of actively shaping how one is to be seen by society when this presentation of self may envelop multiple forms supported by a diversity of technologies. The nature of identity depends on where one is, with whom and what one is doing at the time.

There are many ways to live out being deafened. The process of decision-making associated with being deafened is influenced by what Moore (1994) identifies as the extent of one's personal investment in particular people or associations. Similarly, Dowsett develops the notion of attachment when discussing identification with the Gay Community:

> attachment is not something a person possesses to a greater or lesser degree, but a process of constructing a meaningful daily life within a collectively produced social frame . . . there is no single community; there are only ever-changing dominant cultural forms and identities supported, in some cases, by an increasingly sophisticated urban infrastructure.
>
> (Dowsett 1994: 71)

Sandra and Jan gradually developed personal investments in diverse networks over long periods of time. Carol did not. It is evident then that there is a point to work to, or to avoid, in which a process of personal formation may result in the development of a disability identity that incorporates into one's lifestyle and networks the acceptance or rejection of specific discursive practices. Some people, such as Sandra and Jan, are able to take on specific practices, and involve themselves in new networks wherein they may (or may not) be identified as Deaf, as disabled, as other. If the onset of deafness symbolizes a chasm, a deafness identity symbolizes a light at the end of the tunnel. Central to developing this new identity is the recognition, by deafened people and others, of the experience of heterogeneity that deafness creates; an experience that is not necessarily negative. As Starr (1991: 30) observes, 'Multiple marginality is a source not only of monstrosity and impurity, but of a power that at once resists violence and encompasses heterogeneity.'

Present clinical practices allow little opportunity for deafened people to recognize or work through their experience of multiple selves, contested identity or their multiple encounters with marginality. Clinics work from the assumption that deafened people are only marginalized from hearing culture and that there is an understandable legitimacy in such marginality. From the clinic's perspective, the solution is to assimilate deafened people back into hearing culture. Rehabilitation providers need to examine the presumption that simply because a person is deaf, that they would want to be just hearing people, or that a technology-based intervention (such as the cochlear implant) is necessarily the intervention of first choice. Rather the first point of intervention may be an encounter between the newly deafened person and their network, with people such as Sandra and Jan, coupled with a facilitated introduction to the politics of disability, practice and personal identity.

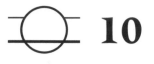 **10**

# Discourse and identity: disabled children in mainstream high schools

## Mark Priestley

The slightest word has an echo far beyond what you can hear;
the smallest deed casts a shadow broader than you can see.

(Zipes 1987: 247)

Language is a social phenomenon. As such, it is embedded within wider social processes and relationships of power. The way we acquire and use language not only reflects our relationship to the wider social world, it also reproduces it. When we speak in terms of gender, race, class, age, sexuality or disability we are also contributing to the production of those same social divisions and categories. Moreover, when we name ourselves, or when others name us within such categories, we too are being produced.

The discussion in this chapter explores some of these issues through the experience of disabled children at two mainstream high schools. The primary data is drawn from informal discussions and participant observation with approximately 20 pupils aged between 11 and 16 (where children's names are mentioned in the text they have been altered). The data was collected as part of the 'Life as a Disabled Child' project, funded through the Economic and Social Research Council's *Childhood 6–16* programme. This project, which focuses on disabled children's own experiences and perspectives, is a collaborative venture between the Disability Research Unit at the University of Leeds and the University of Edinburgh.

There are many parallels between recent developments in childhood studies and disability studies. Both have sought to generate theoretical perspectives on the construction of social inequality and exclusion. Both have been framed within new discourses of individual and collective rights. Both have emphasized the need for participatory research methods that allow excluded voices to be heard (Morrow and Richards 1996; Barnes and Mercer 1997). As Brannen and O'Brien (1995: 737) argue:

What is needed is a social science of childhood which gives central place to the construction of childhoods and their different structural conditions and inequalities whilst at the same time elucidating children's own experiences, definitions and constructions of their daily lives.

Yet there has been relatively little work that explores the intersection between new perspectives on childhood and disability. Much previous research has compounded a view of disabled children as passive, dependent and vulnerable. Moreover, the voices of disabled children themselves have frequently been excluded from the published narratives of this research. As a consequence, such narratives have frequently concealed the way in which disabled children function as social actors, negotiating complex identities within a disabling environment (Priestley 1998).

## Discourse and identity

Disabled children are confronted on a daily basis with ways of speaking about disability that influence their experience and their sense of identity. Negative portrayals of disability abound and disabled children in particular have been subject to institutional discourses of tragedy, medicalization and otherness. Media portrayals and legislative categories often construct disabled children as dependent, vulnerable and 'in need'. From Tiny Tim to *Telethon*, the public discourse of childhood disability emphasizes personal tragedy and vulnerability. These discourses are, in turn, reproduced through daily encounters with other children, with adults and with a variety of institutional contexts.

Thompson (1990) emphasizes the ideological function of language in the creation and maintenance of social relations of power. Such ideology may be conveyed through macro-linguistic strategies, involving whole narratives, or through micro-linguistic practices, in which short phrases and even single words carry ideological significance. As Davies (1989a: 1) puts it, 'in passing language on to children we also pass on a relative entrapment in the social order'. Such discursive practices are evident in many contexts. For example, Knowles and Malukjær (1996) analyse the controlling ideology of children's literature while Waitzkin (1979, 1989) shows how 'structural patterns of domination and oppression' are reproduced in micro-interactions between doctors and patients.

The discourses that disabled children encounter in a mainstream high school, and the discursive categories they acquire in the process, contribute both to their own identity development and to the construction of disability as a social concept. The dominant narratives of 'charity', 'treatment', 'provision' and 'abuse' suggest non-reciprocal processes in which disabled children are more acted upon than acting. They are often stories of passivity, surveillance and confinement (Priestley 1998). However, children are not simply passive recipients. They are also social actors, responding to discursive practices, resisting and reconstructing them to fit their own experiences and priorities. Disabled children in mainstream schools need to continually work out ways of placing themselves within and without the discursive categories of 'disability' and 'special need'. Yet we know relatively little about how this happens in relation to disability.

From a Foucaultian perspective, identity is constructed in two ways. On the one hand, we become known to others through a variety of external disciplines and discourses (many of them institutionally embedded). On the other hand, we make ourselves known through self-knowledge and by speaking about ourselves. In this way, we are both made into, and make ourselves into, social subjects. Shakespeare (1996) develops this approach in relation to disability identity, showing how disabled people have been negatively identified, through dominant discourses, and how they have positively identified themselves, through the development of new discursive spaces and narrative possibilities.

## Becoming known

Within a mainstream high school, disabled children become known through a variety of discourses. Formally, they may become known through statementing procedures and monitoring systems, or through institutional arrangements which differentiate them from other pupils (such as sitting next to a special needs assistant in class, going to a separate 'unit' for certain lessons, being excused from games, etc.). For example, Shelly was conscious that when she had adult support in the classroom, she was separated from normal interactions with other pupils. On these occasions she would sit at a separate desk with the special needs assistant.

*Mark:*   So, do you always have support in class?
*Shelly:*   God, no. I prefer it when I haven't got support because it's more . . . interesting. You can talk to your mates.

In another school, disabled children received much of their support from other pupils. In particular, there seemed to be an established culture of 'helpers' among the children. While this system of support was encouraged by the school, it seemed to be maintained informally by the children themselves. For example, Craig and his non-disabled friend Rachel chatted openly about their relationship. Rachel described how she saw the role of helper:

*Mark:*   So what happens and how do people decide who pushes who? Is it just friends who do it, or does somebody get told to do it?
*Rachel:*   Friends . . . if you've got any, and he has.
*Mark:*   If you've got any?
*Rachel:*   He's got me . . . so he's all right.
[ . . . ]
*Mark:*   So like if somebody was leaving early to go to lunch . . . are they likely to get somebody to go with them?
*Rachel:*   Yeah. We're always late to lessons 'cos we have to get him up in the lift. And if the lift breaks down that's annoying.

*Mark:* What happens if you've got no friends then?

*Rachel:* You're alone [laughs]. You go round on your own, or the dinner ladies help you and get your lunch.

This seemed to suggest that the helper/helped relationship was an informal one worked out among the pupils. However, such relationships can also introduce formal distinctions and hierarchies between disabled and non-disabled children. Rachel sometimes found herself identified as Craig's 'helper' by the staff, drawing her into a more formal role, and thus into a power system which constrains the normal dynamics of peer friendship. There is a sense in which such processes resemble the way that 'informal carers' at home can become formalized through contact with social workers, medical staff and 'care managers' (see Davis 1995).

Informally, disabled children are made known by the way other adults and children in school talk about them, and by the way these references are either accepted or challenged by others. Such differentiation may take many forms. For instance, the classroom observations provided many examples of disabled children being informally exempted from normal disciplinary procedures. In particular, teachers in the mainstream schools seemed less likely to punish disabled children for minor rule-breaking incidents, even where there were clear guidelines for disciplinary action. Two examples help to illustrate the point.

On one occasion, an RE teacher was beginning her lesson with a review of the class homework scores. As she called each name in turn, the child would respond with a score. Those who had not done well, or who had not done the work at all, were severely rebuked in front of the class. Indeed, the teacher seemed unwilling to accept any explanation, no matter how plausible. However, when it came to Emma's turn (the only blind girl in the class), the absence of her homework went unquestioned.

*Boy:* I've got a note.

*Teacher:* You what?

*Boy:* I've got a note.

*Teacher:* Just tell me, 'cos I need to know.

*Boy:* [quietly] My mum was ill and I had to look after her.

*Teacher:* I'm sorry but that goes down as a homework not done ... Kelly?

*Girl:* Four.

*Teacher:* Four? Well I should take that grin off your face. 'Cos the mistakes you made in that homework were classic for somebody that wasn't listening in the lesson ... Nicola?

*Girl:* Fourteen.

*Teacher:* Fourteen ... Emma? Oh, did you do it Emma with someone?

*Emma:* [nervously] No miss, I hadn't had a chance yet.

*Teacher:* Oh right.

There may have been good reason not to question Emma's lack of homework. She may normally have had some assistance with the work and the SEN teacher had been absent the previous week. The teacher's response also conveyed an assumption that Emma could not have produced any work unless she had done it 'with someone', despite the fact that Emma is a competent Braille reader who can produce high-quality written work when she has accessible materials to work from. Emma is a conscientious student and the teacher may have known that she would not miss the work without good reason. However, many of the non-disabled children in the class may also have had good reason for their poor performance (particularly the boy with the note). However, the differential treatment was in keeping with a common discursive practice among staff, who often seemed to regard homework produced by disabled students as more of a bonus than a requirement. As another teacher put it:

*Teacher:*  I shouldn't really say this, but we're not so bothered about the academic side [for the students with learning difficulties]. It's the social side really.

On another occasion, a science teacher was attempting to establish order at the beginning of a class. She had already written the names of two pupils on the board (a kind of 'yellow card' before issuing detentions) when Darren, a teenage boy with Down's syndrome, arrived several minutes late. As the teacher questioned his lateness, the other two (non-disabled) boys urged her to follow the standard procedure:

*Teacher:*    Were you dawdling? [no reply] Were you taking your time getting here? [no reply]
*First boy:*    Write his name on the board miss, go on.
*Second boy:*  Yeah, he were last here miss.
*Teacher:*    I know what to do.

The two non-disabled boys spoke indignantly, conveying a direct challenge to the teacher, urging her to write Darren's name on the board. However, they were also laughing, not at the latecomer but at the teacher, daring her to discipline him in the obvious belief that she wouldn't bother. They did not show any animosity towards Darren himself and they did not seem to be particularly bothered about getting him into trouble. Rather, it was as if they knew the teacher would not punish someone with learning difficulties in front of the class. Ultimately, they were correct. Although the teacher looked embarrassed, and admitted to the class that she knew 'what to do', she never did write Darren's name on the board and the incident went unrecorded. He never did say why he was late or apologize to the teacher.

These brief examples provide some pointers to the way in which disabled children can become differentially constructed within a mainstream school. Children have a keen sense of fairness and the differential application of discipline or punishment rarely goes unnoticed in a classroom. Students with special educational needs are frequently distinguished from their non-disabled peers by formal and informal practices. This kind of ritual, and very public, 'othering' reinforces powerful discursive messages in the minds of pupils. Based on a cumulative experience of small incidents, they begin to build discursive categories of 'special needs' or 'disability'. Without more detailed knowledge, we can only wonder what messages pupils pick up. Disabled children are different? Disabled children can't produce work on their own? Disabled children can't help being naughty? Disabled children don't get told off? Much more work is needed to uncover the ideological significance of discursive practice in schools.

## Making known

As well as becoming known from without, disabled children also make themselves known through their own talk and through resistance to received discourses. For this reason, Allan (1996) argues that we should examine not only the official discourse of 'special need', within its institutional context, but also the 'points of resistance' (Foucault 1976: 95) that children generate for themselves; 'for children with SEN, this would involve looking for evidence of them challenging the identities they are given or opting for alternative experiences' (Allan 1996: 222).

Low (1996: 244) lists a number of resistance strategies employed by disabled college students. These included speaking out, reasoning with others, using humour, being assertive or aggressive, avoiding confrontations, distancing from other disabled students. Davies (1989b: 239) points to various forms of resistance employed by school students (such as laughter and confrontation). However, she suggests that very few of these are 'constructive resistances' because they usually fail to dislodge the oppressive discursive practices to which they are responding. She concludes: 'At most they develop their own discursive practices through which they can accord themselves a sense of self-respect or self-worth, but this "alternate" discourse exists outside the meaning structure recognised and legitimated by the school authorities' (p. 239).

The most obvious resistance among the children was in response to name calling and teasing by other (non-disabled) pupils. Several of the children spoke spontaneously about such incidents. They were also able to talk about their reactions. For example:

*Craig:* Well, there's just this one . . . [older boy]. And every time I go past him [in my wheelchair] he just shouts something like 'run!', or summat.

*Mark:* So how do you feel about that sort of thing?

*Craig:* I put up wi' it the first few times but then I told him to stick it.

Bev (who has learning difficulties) and Emma (who is blind) dealt with such situations in very different ways:

*Bev:* But I've learnt to deal with it me, and if anybody says out very nasty to me, and I'm with anybody who knows 'em, you know, I'll just turn round and smack 'em.

*Emma:* Just ignore 'em.

*Bev:* No, hit 'em, or call 'em it back, they don't like that.

*Emma:*   . . . I just tell 'em to shut up, [inaudible] really nice but.
*Bev:*     I don't. I turn round and smack 'em one.
       [later in the same conversation]
*Bev:*     We've adapted to it haven't we Emma?
*Emma:* Yeah.
*Mark:*   What d'you mean adapted? In what way?
*Bev:*     We get used to it [laughs].
*Emma:* If people swear I just ignore 'em, they shut up, or tell em, or say to
       'em, that's not very nice.

The strategies used by the two girls are clearly very different. There are of course many reasons why different children react in different ways (personality, age, social background, culture, etc.). However, the important point here is that, like other children who spoke about such incidents, they were by no means passive in the construction of their own identities within the school context. These are not the passive, vulnerable children of the Dickensian novel or the socio-medical research literature.

Another important way in which children make themselves known at school is through their choice of peer friendship groups. At school, children are both formed into groups and form themselves into groups. Clustered integration, centrally resourced 'special needs' units and school taxis often bring children of different age, gender, class and race together in impairment-specific situations. Sometimes these groupings form the basis for enduring personal friendships, but for many disabled children in mainstream schools, friendship networks are based on other criteria.

For example, initial observations in one school suggested the existence of a small, impairment-specific friendship group, congregating at break times around the special needs unit. However, it soon became clear that age and gender were the main factors. Although the group always included three or four of the younger visually impaired girls, it never included any of the boys, or the older girls. In addition, other non-disabled girls of a similar age would join the group from time to time. The following extract from a conversation with one of the older girls suggests that age was important to her.

*Mark:*   You don't seem to play with that gang that hang out by the [special
       needs] unit?
*Shelly:* No, I'm older.
*Mark:*   'Cos they all seem to hang out together?
*Shelly:* Yeah, they do.
*Mark:*   Why's that then?
*Shelly:* It's because they're younger I think, and I'm older.

Age is certainly the most institutionalized form of social grouping in schools (since children are clearly divided into year groups, curriculum Key Stages and so on). However, within children's own groupings, gender tends to be a key factor. Although boys and girls do play together at school, they mostly play apart and close friendships are more likely to develop from same-gender interactions (Goffman 1977; Thorne 1993). Race/ethnicity is also important in friendship networks at school, although it rarely takes precedence over age and gender (Schofield 1982).

When priority is given to a child's 'disability' or 'special needs' status this can mask the true complexity of individual identities (Priestley 1998). When asked, disabled children are less likely to see their future selves shaped by disability status as by other social influences (Jahoda *et al*. 1988; Norwich 1997). Indeed, children often choose to reject, accept or redefine identity labels in different situations and at different times (James 1993). Thus:

> We each learn to operate within multiple discourses that are in conflict with each other. Furthermore, we position ourselves, and are positioned differently within each different form of discourse depending on the power and resources that we have at hand.
>
> (Davies 1989b: 239)

The key words here are 'power' and 'resources'. Reflexivity is not unbounded (Giddens 1991) and disabled children are not simply free to 're-invent' themselves at will. More often than not, they are constrained by relationships of power, by disabling environments and by disabling institutional arrangements. However, mainstream school life also provides many opportunities for flexibility and negotiation.

## Negotiating identities

Allan (1996) found that the disabled children she observed did not adopt fixed disability identities or standardized strategies for resistance. Rather, their sense of identity shifted as the result of an ongoing and dynamic process of identification with a number of different discourses. Low's (1996) research with older college students illustrates some of this complexity. Low describes how the students sought to reject the (negative) disabled identities which were imposed upon them by other staff and students. However, in order to negotiate disabling barriers in a mainstream campus, they often found it necessary to revert to a 'disabled' identity. Thus, 'In order to achieve a non-disabled identity, students with disabilities must successfully negotiate a physical environment which in its inaccessibility isolates them from interaction with others, emphasising their disabled identities' (Low 1996: 246).

Allan and Low's analyses provide a good description of the strategies adopted by children in the two schools. On the one hand, the children were categorical in rejecting negative disability labels, especially from other students. On the other hand, they were able to skilfully manipulate disabled identities when they thought it would work to their advantage (e.g. getting out of lessons or avoiding punishment from teachers). The following examples provide a flavour of these strategies.

Anna's weekly English class involved class reading from a set book. Since there was no Braille copy for Anna to read (she had a taped version at home), the objective of the lesson, reading and following the text, was not an option for her. From an educational perspective, this raises issues of curriculum access but for Anna it was not a major problem, since she could avoid doing very much during the lesson.

> I don't know if we're reading or writing today. It looks like a good book though. It's good if you're reading because I haven't got anything Brailled, so I just listen.

> (Anna)

Craig was able to point out physical access problems for wheelchair users in his school. The geography of the school prevented him from getting to certain classes on time. However, he was also able to see how being a wheelchair user could be turned to advantage when arriving late for other reasons.

> 'Cos like another thing that could be better in this school is the access. You see out there [nods to window] there's like three ramps? Well it'd be easier, 'cos like if they just had one like, ramp going from like one place to another. Because if you're down there in [that] area right, you've got to go up all the way up three ramps to get to science, but in [that] area there's like a set of steps that you just go straight up, and you're at science. So basically it takes a disabled person like 15 minutes to get to science, takes everyone else like ... I mean sometimes I do muck about on me way to lessons, but then I just say me chair's slow, you know [laughs].

> (Craig)

During an all day Art project, Michelle was working well on her own. As a result, she had finished most of the task in the first session and was getting bored. During the morning break she had enjoyed talking with her close friend and didn't really feel like going back to the art project. So, using her 'disabled' identity, she tried to get her non-disabled friend out of a maths class until lunch time by asking the teacher for a 'helper'.

*Michelle:*  Miss, can my friend come with me after break?
*Teacher:*  We've already got five helpers in class so I think we're OK as we are.
*Mark:*  [in private, on the way to class] Does your friend come and help you often in class?
*Michelle:*  No, I was bored and I just wanted someone to chat to.

In the classroom, Michelle had taken probably the 'least disabled' role among her peers yet she was quick to adopt a 'disabled' role with the teacher when she thought it might be to her advantage. On this occasion it did not work but it was clearly a strategy well known among the disabled pupils in the school. Back in the Art room, and approaching lunch time, David tried a related ploy.

*David:*  Sir, sir, can we go to lunch early [with a smirk] 'cos we're disabled?
*Ben:*  [scornfully] Disabled?
*Mark:*  What sort of an excuse is that?
*Mike:*  [mimicking David] I'm really, REALLY, disabled [laughs].
*Mark:*  Is that a word you use?

*David:*    Yeah.
*Michelle:*  Yeah, they go early because it takes ages to get there.

David, Ben and Mike were, like Michelle, also happy to play out the 'disabled' role when they thought it would be a successful negotiating tactic with adults (or with each other). However, as the above extract shows, this was invariably done with a high degree of irony and self-awareness. Importantly, all these examples show disabled children as social actors, engaging directly with institutional discourses of disability, and actively reconstituting them to their own advantage.

Bearing this in mind, it is important to be reflexive about the role of the researcher in ethnographic research. For example, the younger boys' apparent bravado may well have been influenced by my presence as a male researcher in a mixed gender group of children. We need to be especially aware of our own part in the story, and sensitive to the ways in which children may change their narratives to take account of our presence. The construction of children, and particularly disabled children, as passive subjects has legitimized falsely-premised claims to objectivity on the part of disability researchers in the past (Stone and Priestley 1996). To acknowledge disabled children as creative social actors is to acknowledge that they will act just as consciously when they are 'being researched'.


## Conclusions

Using the example of gender, Davies (1989b: 1993) describes how children learn to recognize discursive categories that include some people and exclude others. They then participate in various discursive practices that give meaning to these categories. As a consequence, they begin to position themselves imaginatively in relation to such categories and come to recognize themselves as having an identity within them. Moreover, they develop a sense of 'emotional commitment' to category membership and a moral system organized around this sense of belonging. Although Davies argues that our 'sense of who we are' is open to a range of possibilities, she also points out that common discursive practices steer children towards unitary, and mutually exclusive, categories. In this way, she shows how the discursive categories which children encounter at school create males and females as 'opposites' (boys and girls, rather than children). Importantly, these opposing categories also convey, and reproduce, social relationships of power in the wider world. Thus:

> Current understandings of what it means to be a person require individuals to take themselves up as distinctively male or female persons . . . The opposition embedded in the terms is not an opposition of equals, but one in which part of the definition of one is its dominance over the other.

> (Davies 1989b: 234)

Similarly, Iris Young (1990) suggests that notions of 'same' and 'other' are symptomatic of a more generalized preoccupation with conceptual dichotomies – what Adorno (1973) calls the 'logic of identity'. The tendency to classify things which are similar into a category of 'same' generates a logically opposing category of 'other'. In turn, Young argues, such dichotomies become associated with the underlying normative dichotomy 'good/bad', so that 'same' equals 'good' and 'other' equals 'bad'. This process then obscures the richness and plurality of difference.

Disability discourse within schools can create just such pressures on children to identify with one of two logically opposing categories – disabled or non-disabled – which are also hierarchically arranged. For example, there is considerable evidence that children with hearing impairments are subject to powerfully opposing identities of 'deaf' and 'hearing' at a very early age (Erting 1994; Corker 1997). The integration of children with impairments into mainstream high schools has provided many opportunities to blur these discursive boundaries, especially among children themselves. However, the language of 'special need', and the discursive practices used to police it, continue to construct disabled children as the other.

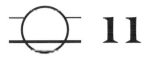 **11**

# Transforming disability identity through critical literacy and the cultural politics of language

**Susan Peters**

## Introduction – the culture of silence

*Voice of a learning-disabled student*
If you found out what they're not good at and put a label on them they would feel real low because you are messing around with their weakness. And no one wants you to play with their weakness because if it is your weakness you can say too much about it.

Worldwide, people with disabilities experience invasion of their disability identity through the practices of labelling and hegemonic language usage detrimental to their images. These practices result in significant negative consequences and barriers to productive living. Many disabled people (particularly youth) internalize labels and language used to inculcate them as passive recipients in welfare-oriented societies. They develop a false consciousness as they internalize the oppressors' image conveyed through language. This cultural invasion leads many disabled people to a silent world of passive acceptance where they adapt to the status quo of a governmental system devoted to their 'welfare' rather than achieve an integrated positive identity from their own lived experiences.

A small, but growing, number of educators have recognized the relevance of Paolo Freire's work with 'illiterate' peasants in Brazil to the problems of 'at-risk' students in urban education settings in North America and other countries where the alienation of students in post-revolutionary and advanced industrial societies has become endemic. Peter Mayo, for example, has provided an excellent critique of Freire's work in a variety of contexts. He arrives at the conclusion I embrace in the context of my own work with disabled youth that 'Freire's method of conscientization through critical literacy can become a vehicle for the consolidation of a new political and social order' (Mayo 1995: 373). While Mayo analyses post-revolutionary contexts in Africa and Latin America, others, such as Ira Shor (1987), have specifically applied Freire's cultural literacy to a variety of North American contexts.

In the context of Disability Studies, education in the USA has, until the current time, embraced a medical model of disability, or a functional limitations model steeped in paternalism. Despite the growing recognition of the 'minority rights' model espoused by disability activists, education has by and large remained impervious to this new paradigm. The pathological view of disability sets up paternalistic social relationships which strengthen the subservient status of disabled people, requires them to be labelled as deficient, and shunts them off to special education classrooms (and even pseudo-inclusive general education classrooms) where they languish in a culture of silence reinforced by a 'banking model' of education. This model views students as empty repositories to be filled with knowledge, but in reality this knowledge amounts to learning required rules of conformity and unproblematized values hidden within a language and discourse of deviance and deficiency. Such 'knowledge' is supposed to accumulate interest and cultural capital for successful participation in a democratic society. However, this form of education too often results in alienation, worsens the literacy problem and school failure, and relegates disabled students to a silent *and silenced* world, where they become what they are perceived as being: incapable, illiterate, dysfunctional and non-productive members of school and society.

Skrtic (1995) has written eloquently about these conditions and their causes. His critique uncovers significant problems with the current situation and is primarily limited to a North American context, but does not go far enough in pointing to concrete solutions, perhaps because Skrtic and other disability rights activists have typically focused on solutions at the systems level. Such critiques and political and legislative solutions largely ignore or sideline the other part of the equation: the potential of socio-linguistic approaches aimed at transforming and empowering disabled *individuals* themselves to take the lead role in effecting change.

## Freire's framework of conscientization and critical literacy

The specific methods of critical literacy I propose rest on a Freirean pedagogical framework of *conscientization*. Essentially 'education for liberation' conscientization is the organized act of educating individuals with emphasis on subject instead of object, or the 'Other'. At its core, conscientization involves praxis – a combination of reflection and action – on the part of individuals, which enables them, singly or collectively, to transform oppressive institutional systems. Conscientization is 'learning to perceive social, political, and economic contradictions, and to take action against the oppressive elements of reality' (Freire 1970: 19). The goals of conscientization have been appropriated by a number of oppressed minorities. For example, Sarah

Lawrence-Lightfoot, writing with regard to the process of liberation for Black people in the USA, describes conscientization as:

> the process of making values and experiences that are most often repressed or hidden, conscious and visible to oneself and others. It has to do with courageously uncovering the pain, making it articulate, reckoning with it and entering it into the public/private discourse. It is an uncomfortable demanding process, requiring both thought and action.
>
> (Lawrence-Lightfoot 1994: 3)

This process of conscientization is arrived at through *critical literacy* – a theory of literacy and voice that uses a language of critique and of possibilities. Critical literacy is a counter-hegemonic pedagogy or discourse practice which puts oppressed people at the centre as cultural agents of change. Through this process, language becomes a cultural/political act with the aim of building self-identities, while at the same time holding the goal of transforming societal attitudes and beliefs that have acted to stifle the cultural identities of disabled people. Critical literacy is the key starting point for developing positive identities of disabled people and achieving its ultimate goal – transforming the social, political, cultural and economic contexts within which individuals live. Conscientization and critical literacy start with the individual and a belief in human agency. Together they constitute a form of educational praxis that includes two stages, where oppressed people with disabilities

- unveil the world of oppression, and through praxis come to know themselves as 'subject' and commit themselves to transformation.
- transform the reality of oppression in their everyday lives, resulting in an educational pedagogy that ceases to belong to the oppressors but becomes a pedagogy of all people in the ongoing process of permanent liberation.

## The application of Freire's framework to disability studies

I first encountered conscientization in application to disability studies in the early 1990s through an analysis of disability rights social movements, in particular the Zimbabwean disabled people's struggle for place and identity through a process of educational praxis outside of educational institutions. Their grassroots formulation of conscientization to transform oppressive political, economical and cultural systems provided the impetus for my realization that these methods ought to be considered more systematically in the context of formal schooling of disabled people. The Zimbabwean appropriation of political conscientization contained links to critical theorists in education such as the work of Habermas (1984 and 1987, concept of communicative action), Vygotsky (1934, 'inner speech', where thought and language coincide in word meaning) and other critical theorists in North America. Further, John Dewey's progressive education movement emphasized teaching and learning in classrooms as a problem-solving and question-posing enterprise, one of the main goals of his approach being to problematize the structural positivism and essentialism inherent in US public schools.

The 'learning disabled' students whom I taught and learnt with, and who are the subject of this chapter, saw their problems as isolation, no sense of community, apathy, and paralysis of thought stemming from a dehumanizing educational bureaucracy and excess of power on the part of educational professionals. Much of this power stemmed from the language used to relegate them to a marginal status within schools and society. Therefore, if we could appropriate a historical/political perspective to develop a dialogue in schools around the 'problem' of disability, then a pedagogical solution to isolation might present itself, leading to active student engagement in learning, a sense of community, and political solidarity. I make several assumptions in arguing for this approach to literacy and social competence. The basis of these assumptions is the dictum 'education is political'. But I will discuss these at the end of this chapter. First, I want to begin at the ground level, with student and teacher voices and the process of becoming engaged in education for transformation as a liberating experience, both personally and politically.

**The Literacy Project**

In 1992, I undertook a literacy project to increase the literacy competence of 40 students labelled as 'learning disabled' in a high school composed almost entirely of African-American students. As a result of our work together over a period of three months, we produced an 'underground' newsletter dealing with the subjects of special education, labelling and conditions at the high school, along with recommendations to improve the school community and learning environment.

The Literacy Project is framed by the five phases of Freire's literacy method, found in 'Education as the Practice of Freedom' (Freire 1973), which are as follows:

1 Participant observation of educators 'tuning in' to the vocabulary universe of the people.
2 Search for generative words at two levels: syllable richness and a high charge of experiential involvement.
3 Codification of words into visual images which stimulate people to emerge as conscious makers of their own culture.
4 Decodification under the stimulus of a coordinator who has become educator-educatee in dialogue with educatee-educators who are no longer treated as passive recipients of knowledge.
5 A creative codification explicitly aimed at action. Students reject their role as objects and become subjects of their own destiny.

Freire's five phases of critical literacy have been variously described and interpreted, and it is worth mentioning some examples. Wallerstein (1987) identifies three phases of a 'problem posing method':

- *listening*, which involves naming/identifying emotional, structural and socio-economic blocks to critical consciousness;
- *dialogue*, which entails coding these identifications in writing, stories, photographs, skits, collages or song;
- *action*, where language practice becomes a means to active transformation.

Students can act on their oppression when they link gaining control of their language to assuming responsible control of their lives. By contrast, Finlay and Faith (1987) condense these phases to three basic processes – which they call investigation (of consciousness), thematization, and problematization. I mention these interpretations here because they can be helpful in understanding the precepts involved in implementing a critical literacy programme. However, in this project, as indicated above, I use the five phases as originally proposed by Freire without adaptation, and to provide a concrete explanation of the process. I argue that this framework can be utilized to simultaneously engage students in learning, improve literacy, and promote awareness through conscientization, leading to educational transformation and to liberation from labelling and the special education paradigm of medical and innate pathological deficiencies.

*Phase 1: Participant observation of educators 'tuning in' to the vocabulary universe of the people*

We began our sessions together in groups of six to seven students for one hour a week. These meetings were informal, involving conversations about what it means to be labelled 'learning disabled'. Students in this phase shared experiences that revealed longings, frustrations, beliefs and hopes about their lives. Mainly, the students expressed the belief that they were unable to read or to write because they were 'LD'. They longed to appropriate the big 'important' words that their 'regular' peers and teachers used to describe them and to turn the tables. They hoped that through literacy they would gain the cultural capital they felt they needed to succeed in life.

We began by deconceptualizing and demystifying the term 'learning disabled', which to them, from their position of 'massified conscientization', seemed to be the root of their problems. Massified consciousness is a hegemonic narrative inculcated through mass media. Here, it refers to the accepted language and usage of labels to characterize individual identity in special education. This was achieved firstly by reading aloud together definitions of learning disability which were taken from textbooks used in introductory university courses on special education, and deconstructing this meaning through conversation. Secondly, I shared with them my own writing about labelling and its social meaning, with the aim of moving from massified to critical consciousness concerning the label 'learning disability'. This writing took the form of a short essay I developed in response to an invitation to participate in a conference of special educators. I was told by the conference organizers that I would be allowed three minutes at the end of a panel discussion on new directions in special education. I was also given the topic, which was to comment on the following poem:

> If I am not for myself, then who will be for me?
> But if I am only for myself, then what am I?
> And if not now, when?

(Author unknown)

I should emphasize that I was the only participant with a disability on the panel or in the audience of several hundred professionals. My participation was a token recognition that the silent voices of disabled people should have a place at the table. I titled my essay 'Distorted Perceptions and Misplaced Altruism', and significant portions of it will be given at length here for two reasons. First, it contains a statement of my own political beliefs which provide a context for a critical understanding of the values that drive educators and are too often hidden. Second, it had a powerful impact on the students in the literacy project and formed the springboard for our subsequent exploration of the possibilities of an alternative world view of disability, especially with regard to their experiences in the context of schooling.

---

*Box 11.1*   Distorted perceptions and misplaced altruism

Education professionals have contributed to distorted perceptions through our professional practice. When a student asks, 'If I am not for myself, then who will be for me?', the question implies that we have not provided adequate alternatives, opportunities and experiences because we have perpetuated the myth that people with disabilities do not belong to society and cannot contribute to the goals of society. We have accomplished this feat through our segregation practices and our paternalistic attitudes. If we really believed that students with disabilities have the potential and the right to equal participation in society, why don't we have more people with disabilities in our own profession? Where are the role models that would encourage our students to achieve a better quality of life? If we had been doing our job, we would see more evidence of our success.

I contend that, underneath it all, we don't really believe that people with disabilities can succeed and excel in our society. Why else would we shelter and protect them from the real world? The very profession that holds the promise of advocating for disabled people, instead conveys an altruism that is ultimately destructive . . . We have segregated students in pull-out and separate programmes based on the rationale of 'the good of the child'. We continue to do so in the face of contrary empirical evidence and civil rights suits, arguing that students are better served in specialized environments and that they must be protected from cruel and insensitive peers. We conveniently forget that Black students were marched to school accompanied by armed guards, faced with adults who threatened their lives. Black students were integrated because segregation is inherently unequal, regardless of the racism they faced in integrated classes. The same standard is not applied to people with disabilities in the name of benevolent humanitarianism. We don't acknowledge that you can't teach a child to swim in the mainstream without putting that child in the water. We have closed the doors to equal opportunity and a free society by segregating students. We are protecting them, not from cruel and insensitive students, but from adults (teachers and professionals) who provide the models from which students take their cue.

What can be done to alleviate the segregation, to change our low expectations for achievement, and to improve the quality of life for people with disabilities? I believe we need to own up to our own distorted perceptions and misplaced altruism. We need to ask ourselves, 'If I am only for myself, then what am I?' To answer this question we need to label ourselves, assess our own potential for achievement, and evaluate our own progress towards our maximum potential as enablers of people who have much to contribute to our society. There are three categories of special education professionals: moralists, rationalists and pragmatists. (Proper labels might be 'morally impaired', 'rationally disturbed' and 'pragmatically handicapped'.) The morally impaired argue that students with disabilities belong in pull-out programmes that 'protect' them from societal mistreatment. The rationally disturbed continue to assess progress or lack of progress ad nauseam while students with disabilities await placement decisions in limbo. The pragmatically handicapped credo can be capsulated in the rallying cry, 'We're not ready yet.' But students are ready . . . one student said, 'I know my abilities and I want to show people what I can do.' There are many other students like this one, and they are not waiting for the pragmatists to decide when we might be ready for them. They are asking the question, 'If not now, when?'

There is a fourth category of professional – social constructivist (societally maladjusted). It is a new category I created for myself because I don't fit into any of the other categories. So far as I know, I'm one of a very low incidence population, but I'd like others to join me. A social constructivist believes there are multiple realities and that truth lies in the eyes and mind of the beholder. Where these truths are distorted by misplaced altruism and 'benevolent' humanitarianism, the social constructivist works to change perceptions, to provide new paradigms. This work requires that labels be destroyed (including those I have created to illustrate my points) and that segregated classrooms be relegated to times past.

Some examples follow of student observations during our conversations, which were subsequently encoded in written form.

All students should be treated the same way.

Do teachers think it is right for you to have your learning cut short?

Everyone has problems and alter-egos to maintain, and mine is to succeed in life and not let anyone else be pulling me down.

I feel that people shouldn't label other people, because they don't like to be labelled themselves. If more people would think about how it feels to be called a name or put in categories, they would know how it feels to be called a name.

If you found out what they're not good at and put a label on them they would feel real low because you are messing around with their weakness.

It makes me feel real angry to hear people talk about other people. It's just not right because I think that the next person is no better than me.

I feel labelling puts so much pressure on you because you have to put up with people calling names, making fun of you.

Following the group's oral reading of this essay with the students in the Literacy Project and the deconstruction of disability definitions in official textbooks, students shared their feelings about their experiences. As a result, we began to respect each other, and to understand the nature of our oppression – the beginnings of tuning in to the vocabular universe of disabled people.

*Phase 2: Search for generative words at two levels: syllable richness and a high charge of experiential involvement*

Students now wanted 'big words' to express their feelings – words that had phonemic richness, phonetic difficulty and a 'pragmatic tone' (implying a 'greater engagement of a word in a given social, cultural and political reality', Freire 1973: 51). These expressions were links between words and the thing it designates. We started by listing the first words that came to mind to describe

*Table 11.1*    Conceptual designations

| Words | Generative/conceptual designation |
| --- | --- |
| school | harsh, arbitrary, uncaring |
| learn | gain knowledge |
| teachers | insincere, didactic |
| fight | altercation, harassment |
| principal | aloof |
| gossip | rumour, malicious |
| judgement | false accusations |
| loss | deprivation |

the school (left column, Table 11.1). Next, we discussed the deeper contextual meaning of these words. Students described some teachers, for example, as standing in front of the room and talking at them, not allowing them to talk. I suggested the word 'didactic', which we looked up in the dictionary. Students felt this was an apt description and appropriated the word for use as a conceptual designation of teachers. We followed this process of a search for conceptual designations for each of the descriptive words we generated (right column, Table 11.1).

*Phase 3: Codification of words into visual images which stimulate people to emerge as conscious makers of their own culture*

In this stage we categorized descriptive words in three areas that encompassed the totality of their schooling experiences:

*What it's like*
great loss-deprivation

*What we do*
curse didactic teaching
fight, harass each other
malicious gossip

*How we feel*
aloof
pessimistic
frustrated
nervous

From this codification, students were establishing critical consciousness, while at the same time learning to read and write.

*Phase 4: Decodification under the stimulus of a coordinator who has become educator-educatee in a dialogue with educatee-educators who are no longer treated as passive recipients of knowledge*

During this phase, we discussed the purposes of reading and writing, the power of language to convey values and beliefs, and who our audience might be. The students decided to write a newsletter to teachers and students. They chose the title *From Our Voice*. Each student wrote individual contributions that progressed through several drafts until they felt satisfied with the results. After each draft, students shared their writing and solicited feedback. We used a simple method I introduced called TAG: Tell what you like, Ask questions, Give feedback. Some students chose long essay formats, some chose short poetic 'rap' forms. All of their writing conveyed their sense of developing consciousness in powerful literary images. At this phase, the students put the words in phase 3 together to express their developing consciousness in literary images. For example:

Here at Wildcat City we feel that we need to stick together as a school. Many students are ready to leave the Wildcat's City. Wildcat administrators need to be less aloof in the school. They need to take more time to smile.

Some of the teachers are didactic. They talk all day but you still don't know what to do, so you want to go to sleep on them and they get mad. But how can I stay awake with someone that I don't know what they're talking about?

Northwestern is a big enormous school. But we have a lot of people who like to gossip about people, and at other times they have false accusations to make about some people, when already most people have the most pessimistic side of things.

The students' literary signatures gave final testimony to their development of positive personal identities. They signed each of their compositions with an African name chosen to convey who they were as an individual. Toya signed her essay entitled 'Can't Miss Reality' with the name *Mashingaidze*, a Shona word she chose for herself which means Complex Person. Greg chose *Mandivamba*, a word meaning Practical/No Nonsense for his essay, entitled 'Don't Label Me If You Don't Know Me'. Tawana became *Dekesai*, The Laughing One, in her rap song, 'Beaten Up'.

*Phase 5: A creative codification explicitly aimed at action. Students reject their role as objects and become subjects of their own destiny.*

At this stage, students were eager to make recommendations to alleviate and/or transform their experiences of school as oppressive. These recommendations were published in their newsletter, along with their writing about labelling and their school experiences. The students made 12 recommendations (Box 11.2) in all, many of which were implemented.

---

*Box 11.2*    Sample of student recommendations

- More freedom around school. Right now we're treated like caged animals. If you treat people like caged animals then they'll respond like that.
- We need more school spirit.
- Students should have more say. Especially for seniors, more say in decisions that affect them, like the decision to have graduation ceremonies at another school instead of our own.
- The administration should think of students in a positive way. Don't make wrong assumptions.
- Teachers need to take time out to discuss the class work; we need to understand more about our work.

---

In its first year, several editions of the newsletter were published. I continue to publish the newsletter each year in my course packet for the university-level course I teach, *Diverse Learners in Multi-Cultural Perspective*. In course evaluations, students comment on the powerful impact these students' voices have had in changing their perceptions of learning disability. But most significantly, through this Literacy Project African-American youth labelled as learning disabled developed a critical consciousness of the nature of their oppression. They developed the ability to analyse, problematize (pose questions) and ultimately to put into words a plan of action to affect the realities of school that shaped their lives. Surrounded by historical and political forces that devalued and dehumanized them, they were able to emerge from their status as object (passive, silenced recipients of the inequities and injustices of a dehumanizing system of special education) and to transform their disability identity to active subject.

## Conclusions: the teacher as educator-educatee and the cultural politics of language

In developing an educational process of conscientization that focuses simultaneously on both literacy and social/political competence, I appropriate five basic assumptions from Paulo Freire about education. I believe that these assumptions should form the core beliefs of educators who work with disabled students.

1  Education is an act of love and courage. It is not a paternalistic love that reveals a disrespect for student capabilities. Nor is it a guilty love based on perceived innate inequalities of capabilities. It is an 'armed love' that promotes self-confidence, self-discovery and self-worth. It is armed with the courage of convictions that reveal themselves in a 'radicalization' of education involving increased commitment to the position one has chosen. 'It is predominantly critical, loving, humble, communicative, and therefore a positive stance' (Freire 1973: 10).
2  Education is not neutral. Curriculum and instruction are a political-pedagogical process. Despite special educators' objective pretences (cloaked in standardized assessments, medical labels and mandated referral procedures), the process of becoming learning disabled is, in fact, a political act (Peters 1996). So is the content taught once one has been labelled. 'One teaches how to think through teaching of content. Neither can we teach content by itself as if the school context in which this content is treated could be reduced to a neutral space where social conflicts would not manifest themselves' (Freire 1993: 24).
3  Literacy/language, comprehension and communication are inseparable. Language is linked to power and ideology. This is never more apparent than in special education, where the label becomes the person. All decision-making and subsequent actions derive from the language used to describe

a person who is considered disabled. Special education, and the language used within its discipline, communicate a medicalization of disability that is all-powerful, with oppressive consequences.

4 Education is dialogical and initiated from students' world view. We must begin at the level where people are, respecting the values, knowledge and language of students. The awakening or development of a critical consciousness requires an active, dialogical educational programme. Through dialogue, a person becomes consciously aware of his/her context, and he/she becomes politicized (Freire 1973: 56).

5 Education is a dialectical relationship between reflection and action, or what is called praxis. As Freire asserts, 'Nobody becomes an educator on Tuesday at four in the afternoon.' For teachers as well as students, education is a continuous development through reflection on practice, followed by action, which in turn leads to further reflection. A necessary feature of praxis is dialogue.

From my experiences as educator-educatee in this Literacy Project, I gained a new language to describe students labelled as learning disabled. In a forthcoming work, I provide an in-depth discourse analysis of these students' narratives – my literary product of our Literacy Project. Contrary to the overwhelming literature on students with learning disabilities that characterizes these students as at-risk, failing, deficient and unable to meet standard expectations in the regular classroom, I found them to be very resilient. I describe them as street-wise philosophers, image makers and jazz improvisationists.

As philosophers, students saw their task in school as maintaining their self-respect. As one student put it, my task is 'to succeed in life and not let anyone else be putting me down'. They feel a deep sense of injustice: 'It's just not right [being put in a special ed classroom] because I think that the next person is no better than me.' Many of the students' responses to being perceived as LD ('loco-dummies') reveal an inner strength buoyed by anger. As one student put it, when people put her down, 'I come to reality and say, "Ain't nobody perfect. You're learning like everybody else."' This inner dialogue displays a self-encouragement which shows through frequently in all students' writing and conversation. Their street-wise philosophy epitomizes itself in one student's admonition: 'Times are going to get hard, but look to the top. Never give up and you'll make it.' Overall, these students' street-wise philosophy reveals a great deal of strength in the face of psychological violence to their images. Their outlook uncovers the thought processes by which students develop and maintain self-respect. But how do they outwardly manage their relations with other students and teachers in school?

As image-makers, students perform a juggling act to manage their relations with other students and teachers. One students provided a telling insight on the ability to juggle the consequences of being labelled learning disabled: 'Labelling makes you one of two things: weak or strong.' From the students' perspective, turning the tables on professionals who ascribe labels to them would lead to significant changes: 'If you found out what they're not good at and put a label on them they would feel real low because you are messing around with their weakness. And no one wants you to play with their weakness because if it is your weakness you can say too much about it.' Class schedules have to be juggled, 'blowing your cover' has to be managed. One student asks, 'Let's say what if they found out [I'm in special ed]? Would they still be my friends? Would they still go to the park with me? Or would they just blow my cover and tell everyone I was in special ed?' He decided not to take the risk, so that 'it was very important that I kept my secret to myself'.

As jazz improvisationists, students with learning disabilities epitomize resilience. Many students' thoughts about being singled out from their peers for special attention are characteristic of musical rhythms and genre. For some students, school seems like a march or a hymn with the same chorus: repetitious and slow. 'Some teachers have us learning out of the same book year after year, then we never have the time to learn that much out of a regular book.' Acutely aware that they are out of step with general education classes, others find a lack of harmony, an out-of syncness: 'Say (for example), if we both had the same book and they [regular education students] would be on page 167 and we would be on page 66 . . .' This type of improvisation creates discord. it is more like a cacophony of sound – an orchestra with no maestro, a song script with no regular beats per measure. Still other students talk about special attention in ways reminiscent of solo performances within a main theme. 'I figured I needed help with maths so I would learn my times tables and get out – that's it!' What students are asking for is learning that has a regular beat, but a faster tempo and which improvises while maintaining harmony. Essentially this requires a musical script where no part is left out, but solos are encouraged, and the range of octaves is unlimited. They want school to be a jazz session: creative, challenging, spiritual, collectively harmonized.

These descriptions are my socio-linguistic contribution to answering the culture of silence and to beginning the task of critical conscientization for myself and for others who read this work. I believe that there is a legitimate role for scholars as activists – activists of the intellect. In the spirit of Paulo Freire's problem-posing educational pedagogy, I ask a final question: who among us is ready to take on the challenge that *Hazvizikamwi* (The Caring One) poses in her essay, 'How I Feel about Special Education': why not give us more learning things?

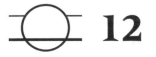 **12**

# Talking 'tragedy': identity issues in the parental story of disability

**Dona M. Avery**

> If there is a Devil, I would sell my soul tomorrow and go happily to Hell smiling all the way to take Michael's [disability] away. After all, I have been there already.
>
> (V—)

Faustian responses to physical disability, or bargaining with the Devil, are not uncommon; our novels and films, religion, art and myths are replete with images of the tortured body, the body distorted by pain, the Picassoesque figure that cries out in anguish and terror. But less often explored is the psychic pain caused by the disability experience, the effects of the social construction of stigma that situate the anomalous body as subaltern. The above quote from the mother of a disabled boy, for example, is representative of the parental impulse to bargain for 'normalcy' for their disabled children; in the mother's view, her son's inability to walk is the most disabling effect of his condition. She goes on to say,

> If there was a cure, if there was a pill, if there was a trade off . . . I would trade my [mobility] for his in a second.
>
> (V—)

Wishing for a magic pill; bargaining with the Devil or with God, to atone for one's child's 'misfortune' – these are common parental responses to what Kenneth Burke calls 'the socialization of losses'. The verbal and symbolic reminders of unmarked-beautiful-healthy-intelligent-'regular' children are ubiquitous in our culture, for society 'privilege[s] strength, beauty, and health over frailty, deformity, and illness' (Rinaldi 1996: 821). Thus, when a newborn is diagnosed with Down's syndrome, cerebral palsy, cystic fibrosis or spina bifida, its parents may grieve for their personal loss (the dreamed-for, hoped-for, 'perfect' child that was not born to *them*). Whereas most parents take personal gratification in compliments of their children – for 'the child is at once outside *them* and of *them*' (Burke, quoted in Gusfield 1989: 297) –

parents of children with disabilities may take personal blame for their less-than-perfect 'production', as if they had 'contaminated' the race. Appropriating the child's 'flaws' as being of their own design, the parents are thus compelled to atone for their 'sin'; and it is from the depths of this guilt that pacts are conceived with the Devil. A journey underground seems preferable to witnessing (what the parent may perceive as) the agonizing life to which her child has been condemned. Most of our cultural understanding of the parental response to disability is heard through doctors' voices, in texts that presume to diagnose, prescribe and thus naturalize the 'mourning' stages parents are reported to undergo when their children are born, or become, disabled (see, for example, Gliedman and Roth 1980; Buscaglia 1983; Mittler 1995; Simons 1997). There is a dearth of published autobiography by parents who candidly explore the socially derived guilt or shame attached to disability. What is more readily available are parental narratives-cum-eulogies that tend to focus on a 'brave child who died too young'.

Where is the parental story of living with what Goffman (1963) calls the 'courtesy stigma', a phenomenon of the gaze that not only judges the differently embodied Other, but endows entire families with the stigma of disability? Where does this tale of 'peripheral prejudice' appear, with its insight into the shifts in a parent's autobiographical cohesion when former notions of the body and 'normalcy' collide after learning one's own child is disabled? This story is, like all personal narratives of disability, 'hard to tell', as Zola (1993) admits; but to share such story with the world is to 'challenge the invisibility that segregation [promotes]'; to silence story 'is to accept invalidity' (quoted in Couser 1997: 213–14). Whereas Zola's call for story is addressed to persons with disability, though, inviting them to publish, to dialogue with the public, I am interested in how disability itself is constructed, and in the linguistic choices parents make as they story themselves and their disabled children, in conversations with each other. The oral discourse of disability is a socio-cognitive territory that has gone largely unexplored; getting together to co-construct a disability or a parenting story has been exceedingly difficult for those living the disability experience, because of social and geographical segregation, transportation difficulties and time constraints. Thanks to advances in computer technology, and access to the Internet, most of those barriers dissolve in cyberspace, where story is now heard 24 hours a day. We are learning that community need not be 'a geographical or demographical or empirical entity' (Miller 1993: 91); and that technology is 'an important social feedback loop'. For scholars, the Net is a 'living database' (Rheingold 1993: 180).

The paradox presented for an analysis of any disability-specific conversation exchange, of course, is that manipulated studies are disabled by the very guilt/shame response that is revealed in the unselfconscious discourse, so that attribution or speaker identity is forfeited. Therefore, for purposes of this paper, I have protected the anonymity of the sources.

As parent of a young man who has a disability, I joined an electronic 'list-serv' whose members are parents new to the disability experience; and after more than a year as participant-observer in this community, I have come to 'know' some of the 250 members. I recognize the constitutive rules of this community, and am able to offer an interpretation of speaker/writer intention and hearer/reader effect, as disability is storied and identities co-constructed within the group. This chapter, then, is an interpretation of stories that I consider to be exemplary of some of the identity issues that commonly haunt parents of disabled children. Using Burke's (1969) 'dramatistic lens' to reveal motive, and employing his theory of guilt and redemption, I hope to contribute to our understanding of the ways in which secrecy and socialized guilt keep oppression in place for the disability culture – just as secrecy and shame enabled the maintenance of other systemic acts of oppression, such as slavery (Equiano 1972; Jacobs 1987) or the Nazi regime, as Burke himself has described.

The disability story of parents needs to be heard; it will inform our knowledge of 'how people come to adopt stories' (Fisher 1972: 235), as well as shed light on the epistemology of 'difference'. Most importantly, the act of telling one's story is a crucial first step toward what bell hooks has called a 'coming to voice'. Because 'illness and disability are deeply embedded in the social world', as Kleinman claims (1988:186), communities (both virtual and physical) have the potential to re-story and restore self within larger society. If we become more aware of the language we use in story, we may also uncover further ways to redefine disability which add to the framework of the social model.

## Guilt, God and the morality play

Disability calls 'for Story' (Frank 1997), and many a newly disabled person has been compelled to write 'a way through disability', while simultaneously 'righting' the self-image, after sudden illness or injury has cognitively deterritorialized the author from the land of 'normalcy'. Identity reconstruction is no less crucial for the parent who finds herself cast in the disability play: she, too, seeks to resolve the dramatic conflict, to 'reconstitute and repair ruptures between body, self, and world' (Williams 1997: 210, 211). Of the 311 electronic conversations held in the electronic performance of the parents' disability story, in the space of one month's time, a Christian-guilt motif appeared in no fewer than 56 subject-lines, representing more than one-sixth of the total topics discussed. The seven originating messages of the 'guilt' story that garnered 56 replies were:

| Originating message | number of replies |
| --- | --- |
| God/guilt | 3 |
| Guilt and all that | 9 |
| Guilt and blame | 5 |
| Guilt and God | 4 |
| Guilt and relationship with God | 21 |
| Guilt/blame | 6 |
| Guilt | 7 |

The 'chaining' effect that compelled such heavy response to the notion of guilt would suggest a deep parental investment in our culture's conflated ideologies in the areas of 'good' parenting and 'perfect' children. It seems clear that we parents tend to situate our children's disability as personal punishment. Simons (1997: 11) substantiates this claim when citing a parent who says, 'I feel like God abandoned me. I feel like I must have done something wrong and now he's punishing me.' Parents blame themselves, moralize and judge themselves, and turn to God in hopes of relieving their psychic pain caused by disability in the family. Note that the issue here is not solely the physical pain that an impairment might be causing the child, for the three uses of the personal pronoun 'I' in the above citation, as well as the implicatures of 'abandonment', 'wrong' and 'punishment', clearly connote a moral imperative that has less to do with the child's duress than with the parent's attitude toward disability. Likewise, the case of the mother who fantasized about a 'magic pill' and a pact with the Devil (as trade-offs for her son's inability to walk) suggests a parental obsession with 'normalcy' as the privileged goal for her child.

Many similar utterances that appear in the electronic corpus seem to replicate what Daniell calls the 'Dear God' letters of recovering alcoholics (1994: 242). Daniell sees therapeutic value in the 'bargaining' letter (a genre she calls 'Composing as Power'); but I wonder if the writing is not motivated more by an impulse to confess, or to plead for redemption. The 'Dear God' letter of the recovering alcoholic appears to be shaded in sorrow, as the author regrets the shame he or she has brought upon the family through substance abuse. In repentance, the letter writer seeks God's help in restoring the family, taking personal blame for their unhappy fate. Through the same lens of guilt and shame we might perceive the bargaining letter of the mother who is willing to go to Hell, if it would atone for her son's inability to walk. Her message, too, is 'guilted' throughout; but what are the parallels between alcoholics and parents of disabled children? If there is social, moralistic blame attached to overindulgence (that is, the alcoholic is morally inferior for being unable to 'control' the physical impulse toward drink), there may be a similar moralizing response to disability, for its suggested lack of bodily control. The 'shame' in either case would be attendant on societal response, the act of stigmatizing. As Burke claims, where there is action, there is drama, and 'if drama, then conflict; if conflict, then victimage' (quoted in Gusfield 1989: 46).

Do parents of disabled children self-inscribe as victims? This is not revealed in the published literature, for such an admission would violate the 'good' and selfless parent role. But when a parent posits her child as victim, and suffers vicariously the social 'stain' she perceives to be attendant on disability, the parent's autobiographical coherence is fractured by *dissoi logoi*, a scrambled collection of competing, contesting 'truth claims' that frame our culture's disability story. The parent is an adult, after all, usually has been reared, 'normalized', and assimilated into a culture whose 'body' language reveals what Burke calls 'a perfection obsession': the insistence that medicine or science is capable of 'fixing' every bodily flaw, 'correcting' every anomaly. This 'telos of

cure' has led to the belief that the body can be 'cosmeticized' and aestheti-
cized and even cloned, to perpetuate culturally defined standards of 'ideal'.
But disability defies medicine, forces us to recognize the vulnerability of the
body, and evokes for parents a range of emotions that, to quote one author,
include 'terror', 'panic' and 'a sense of foreboding' (Simons 1997: 5). If identity is influenced by the forces of language (Dirksen and Bauman 1997: 321),
each conversation of 'tragedy' and each 'victim'-ization of our children chips
away at our own self-esteem: we have produced 'damaged goods' and must
share in the 'spoiled identity' of our children. I have had babysitters refuse to
care for my son because his disability might be 'contagious'; and when he was
captive in a 'special' school for the 'handicapped', I forfeited 'normalcy' as
well, because all my friends were parents of kids in 'regular' schools, and
there was no common story we could share. It does not help that perfect
strangers ask us what is wrong with our child, or ask us about the nature of
our child's problem. It does not help that the media inscribe our children as
'patients', 'victims' and 'sufferers'; or as being 'confined' to wheelchairs.

## The 'Dear Diary' confession

Rather than seek a heavenly audience for the 'Dear God' letter, the parents'
community that converses in cyberspace may perceive the computer screen
as a postmodern diary, a repository for spontaneous story shared with a face-
less, unknown reader. The 'Dear Diary' letter is, in this respect, reminiscent of
stories shared with priests who, cloaked in the anonymity of the confes-
sional, absolve the speaker of guilt. One mother's late-night posting to the
listserve exemplifies the type of cyber-confession or 'Dear Diary' entry in its
soliloquizing tone:

> *Subject: feeling very sad*
> Yesterday was another slap in the face! A day that tells you wake up, and
> stop pretending that your child will be mobile . . . I have had so much
> hope for Erin, you know kinda like a full balloon that slowly deflates
> with each piece of bad news. Right now I'm looking at a power wheel-
> chair that the hospital loaned Erin yesterday. I think, 'what is this doing
> in my house? my child doesn't need this!' Well it wouldn't be here if she
> didn't. Does anyone know what it is like to see someone put your child
> in a chair for the first time?
>
> (S—)

Upon first glance, the intended audience for this message would appear to
be other parents of disabled children whom this mother has 'met' online. It
seems to be a plea for communal support or a request to begin a dialogue that
will result in collective meaning-making or 'redemption'. The writer's use of
the pronominal form of address ('you know'), as well as her direct question to
'anyone', indicate that this mother has actual readers in mind; this has the
markings of a social act, motivated from the need to share story too difficult to

bear in isolation. The mother seeks feedback, 'something to measure against, to lean against ... [provide] fellowship and comfort' (Rheingold 1993: 20).

However, the mother also speaks of herself in the second person ('a day that tells you ...'; and 'stop pretending that your child will be mobile '), which situates this message as a solitary speech event that Burke would describe as 'an "I" addressing its "me"' (Rinaldi 1996: 832). In this double-voiced utterance, the mother's exhibits the genre of writing that Frank calls the 'chaos' narrative, which 'imagines life never getting better . . . [and reveals] vulnerability, futility, and impotence' (Frank 1997: 97). The use of passive voice and other linguistic clues in such narratives demonstrates identity fractures such as depersonalization and detachment from the body (Rinaldi 1996: 824, 827). And there is a circularity, rather than the linear and chronological ordering of most stories. (Note the mother's switching from 'yesterday' to 'now' and back to 'yesterday'.) Aside from exhibiting such dislocation of space and time markers, the chaos narrative also uses metaphor or analogy ('like a full balloon that slowly deflates') and the past perfect tense ('I have had so much hope ...'). The writer in chaos additionally makes frequent use of the impersonal, detached 'it'-cleft ('it is like ...') (Davis and Jeutonne 1997: 108), which the mother's message above repeats twice. Following Biber's work on the linguistic uses of 'it', this may indicate her detachment from a reality that no longer provides perception-guidance or focus for her (Davis and Jeutonne 1997: 91).

But what is the 'it' that makes her so distraught? The linguistic choices made in telling this disability story of a child's first wheelchair offer specific contextualization cues. 'Slap in the face' seems to imply shame or at the very least, chagrin; while the declarative phrases 'wake up' and 'stop pretending' – in this speech community – signify that the fantasizing and bargaining stages of disability recovery have ended. The mother has been confronted by the worst possible scenario: the child will be 'wheelchair-bound', and dreams of 'normalcy' are forever out of reach. The 'bad news' to which the mother refers, and the 'it' signifier in 'Does anyone know what it is like to see someone put your child in a chair for the first time?' – these are references not to 'the chair' (which recalls the notion of finality itself, as in 'electric chair'), but rather to the act, the putting of the child in the dreaded symbol of disability, the indictment of the child as not-normal. The 'it' that most troubles these parents of children with disabilities (and the majority of our culture, perhaps) is only symbolized by the wheelchair; the stigma that the wheelchair represents is what is abhorred.

I suggest, then, that it may be societally induced shame that distorts such parents' identities, rather than personal guilt over having genetically produced a child who may need tools such as wheelchair, cane, hearing aid, or a synthesized-voice computer. These tools are meant to enhance the child's life; but for society they have become more salient markers of alterity. The cognitive implications that are conferred upon these tools implies a semiotic connection with hospitals or institutions, reinforcing the stigma of incapacitation.

I remember my son's first wheelchair. For nearly five years, I squished him into strollers and heaved his heavy body from the stroller to the car seat, and we managed. I delayed that first wheelchair at any cost, because it meant the end of my dream that he would some day walk. But five minutes after a therapist 'put' him, sentenced him, to that chrome-and-rubber monster-maker, he was doing wheelies in the hospital hallway. He was enjoying freedom, mobility and agency, for the first time; like a teenager with his first car. There is no shame in that, and if I felt any guilt, it was because I had deprived him of this independence for so long, due to society's definitions of normalcy.

### The Rorschach test of parenting: seeing one's child where society sees a patient

Another understudied phenomenon of electronic discourse is the preponderance of iconic expressions. The question mark and exclamation point, for example, occur in multiples, in the virtual examples of 'chaos' narratives posted by parents of children with disabilities. The frequency of 'Wh—' questions such as 'Why . . .?????' and 'What . . .????' suggests the confusion that surrounds an identity shaken by disability in the family. If it is true that language is used in order to 'run order through chaos' (Daniell 1994: 245), the way in which the chaos story is punctuated needs to be included as we study disability's power to punctuate lives. These symbolic cues, seen so frequently in cybermessages, can be more revealing – are more revealing – than even the verbal or physical cues of our material environment (Rheingold 1993: 180–1). For instance, in many subject lines and at various points of the messages, the '!' emoticon is lined up like pieces of artillery (e.g. 'Tears!!!!'), indicating the writer's defensive manoeuvres against grief or guilt or other aspects of disability. Just like the war metaphors that Sontag (1978) uses in describing a battle with cancer, the multiple exclamation point reminds us that disability places one's 'core cultural values *under siege*' (Frank 1997: 50) (italics added); and whole threads of conversations may situate the discourse superstructure as war strategies against the enemy: the disabled, 'traitorous' body.

Such conflations of body and battle, when compounded by the artillery and tactics proffered by medicine, may perpetuate in families with disability the 'telos of cure' that permeates the dominant culture. 'I would do anything for a cure for Michael', vows the mother (V—) quoted above, who would make a pact with the Devil if her son could only walk. The trouble is, there are no cures for the disability that this virtual community experiences; and that knowledge has propelled these parents to become medical experts themselves, sharing story and tips, never ceasing in their quest for a new 'fix'. In this sense, the members form a 'knowledge capital' that cannot be found in any medical office or teacherly text; the parents are the experts, the community functions as 'an online brain trust representing a highly varied accumulation of expertise' (Rheingold 1993: 13). On the other hand, if the language of the experts frequently replicates the medicalese heard in exchanges with doctors, if parents make the language of the 'whitecoats' their own (Frank 1997: 141), the vocabulary spoken in the family home might serve to reinforce the inscription of the disabled child as a 'patient', and might promote a 'custodial' view of disability, as exemplified in the media (Braithwaite 1991: 2). Casual and constant use of terminology such as apraxia, scoliosis, rhizotomy, hypotonicity, hydrocephalus shunt, AFOs, Botox, Tefra, Efalex, SDR, CE, AHC, physiatrist, orthotics and ketogenic – which come 'naturally' to these online parents – may have adverse effects upon the child: 'there is danger of personal devaluation' (Phillips 1990: 851).

Adding to this danger is the tradition whereby most parents add a frank, diagnostic 'tagline' to each electronic posting, identifying their child in conjunction with his or her disability and, occasionally, supplying a notation of the date the child's disability was diagnosed, or a surgical anniversary. These virtual IDs do several things: they serve, first of all, to situate the parent as a member of the group – knowing the vocabulary is one's badge of membership; the tradition also serves to inform other online members, particularly the new initiates, of the parent's expertise in one or more specific areas of disability knowledge, thus inviting parents of children with similar disabilities to open, or join in, a dialogue. The language we use (to name, to narrate) and the words we choose (in interpreting, in identifying) are also social tools that help speaker/writer and hearer/reader bridge the gap between Self and Other so as to be understood, to be known. However, the e-mail tags that use Latinate terms for a child's disabling conditions may also serve to wrap up the child's story, and ontologically enclose him or her like a specimen in a butterfly collection. To be known as 'Tommy, spastic athetoid, 6 years old' seems to reduce the child to an inventory of physiological elements; the child becomes a science project, discussed and measured and medicalized even beyond the boundaries of the doctor's surgery, where most children with disabilities spend far too much time as it is.

Parents of children who are disabled at birth are hardly to blame for their obsession with the terminology of illness, however, for they were initiated into 'tragedy talk' right there in the maternity ward, and continue to be socialized in the hospital industry from then on. Dialoguing with doctors, therapists, rehab specialists, pharmacists and salespeople for rehab equipment – these are discourse communities that speak only in medicalese, and that absorb inordinate amounts of the parents' time. But even if it were possible to eliminate the Latinate terminology from our everyday discourse, the medical world guides our lives. Our societal structures, even the smaller social groups such as family, are 'enacted, instituted, legitimated, [and] confirmed . . . by text and talk' (Fairclough and Wodak 1997: 266). If disability calls for medical treatments, the various medical communities will influence the parents' language, not only as to what stories we tell, but also as to how each story is presented and how it is interpreted. Story 'mediates between the individual's personal experience and shared social norms', as Johnstone claims (1990: 129–30), and our world view is one prescribed by medical authorities.

With this in mind, I suggested to the virtual parents' community that we re-story ourselves by taking a more positive stance toward disability, by altering the linguistic preference for pathos, by restructuring an 'overmedicated' vocabulary, and by resisting dialogue of bodily shape and skin, flesh and form altogether. As Allport noted some 50 years ago, our culture's language is already replete with a 'word fetishism' for the human anatomy, and to reduce prejudice, there must be 'a large measure of *semantic* therapy' (quoted in Eschholz *et al.* 1982: 219, italics added). What neither Allport nor other behavioural scientists would mention, however, is that meddling in semantics is all right for the masses, but the 'experts' were empirically rigid. There was an established hierarchy even within the virtual community of parents, of which I was not aware. No extensive overhaul of the group-story could be undertaken without removing the resident doctor from his virtual throne. The 'tragedy' of disability, I have come to understand, is not only in our language, or in the way we story the body; it is embedded in our reification of the medical field.

Dr X, the self-appointed medical authority for our virtual collective, maligned me for seeking to disrupt the status quo by narrating an anecdote that sutured most members into the drama through its rich, community-specific symbolism and its rhetorical magic. My call for change reminded him, as he told the listserv readers, of an incident involving a 'foxier-than-thou woman in her totally stretchy come-f***-me dress', driving a '$50,000 Saab Turbo'. The woman 'stole' the only 'handicapped' parking space, even as Dr X and his disabled son pulled into the parking lot of a local pharmacy, to pick up a prescription. He watched the woman climb out of her car ('major hair and nails and about 10 lbs of jewelry'); then he hailed a policeman to give her a ticket. Later, the woman returned to the scene and, realizing what had happened, 'went ballistic', accusing the DOCTOR (he used capital letters) of being disrespectful to HER. Next, the woman began crying, 'Nobody ever talks to each other anymore!' The policeman berated her for parking in a restricted space.

The story repeated here is lifeless, but told with Dr X's well-known elo-quence, it had a life of its own. Even to the uninitiated reader, the story would have seemed witty, descriptive, entertaining – but without much connection to the situation at hand. There was a transparently obvious misogynistic tone to the story, which might even have deflected the in-group's communicative act of persuasion. To those of us with personal knowledge of the disability experience, though, there were ethical appeals and 'good reasons', as linguist Wayne Booth (1994) would say, that were master strokes in winning the members back to the doctor's version of 'truth'. The motive for the story may be clearly interpreted from Burke's (1969) dramatistic pentad:

1 The act is the wilful violation of the good doctor's lawful parking space in the 'handicapped zone' (since his disabled son was in the car, he felt he'd earned it). Literal translation: I had violated his 'space', and had intruded on his domain, with the intent of insurrection.

2 The scene is the parking lot of a pharmacy, keeper of medicine for his son (and all our sons and daughters) who were helped by, kept alive by, the magical concoctions of doctors.
3 The actor, ostensibly, is the policeman, who enforces society's decree that the disability community has rights to special parking spots.
4 The agency, though, is the basic, methodical, good-conquering-evil manoeuvre: the doctor rights a wrong, by using the Law.
5 The purpose of the doctor-and-policeman ticketing the guilty woman was to punish the offender and thereby maintain the 'sacredness' of the handi-capped parking privilege, so that no one with disabities (or their parents) would again be violated.

As parents who have, universally, perhaps, experienced the same frustra-tion of seeing a non-disabled person take advantage of a parking spot near a shop, members of the listserv were likely to identify with this story. Our chil-dren's needs (medicine, parking spots, the Law) are top priority for each of us, and the insensitive woman who parked illegally was clearly the villain. Using the symbolic handicapped parking space as a 'God term', the doctor interpellated us all into the drama of right and wrong, even as he used the magic of story to entertain us. As a face-saving strategy, the narrative works brilliantly: the parent/doctor recovers the traditional 'sick role' for his child, and situates himself as hero. Readers would therefore equate the intrusive, unlawful woman driver with me – thereby discounting my suggestion that we tell our story ('Nobody ever talks to each other anymore!') with less focus on medicine.

Most parents reading this online fable may have missed the sleight-of-hand as the magician displayed his wit and symbolic forte. But noting the emphasis on the agency/purpose 'ratio' of rhetorical force to the story, the motive (Burke would say) was mysticism, a tool of oppression used by hege-mony. Freire would concur, for he has argued that the magic of language leads people to accept their condition, to resign themselves, rather than ques-tion societal boundaries and limitations (Covino 1995: 703). When one's autobiographical story seems beyond solution, when we are confounded by things we cannot control, it is to magic that we look for resolution; or we bar-gain with mystical entities – God or the Devil – for redemption or atonement of guilt. Meanwhile, we take the word of medicine as a guide to living and to story. Parents of the group-disability story may take the ideas forwarded by a persuasive speaker, adopting his story for their own, perhaps; and with each utterance of the speaker, 'the audience is moved to remake the substance of its identity into a state of oneness or consubstantiality with the speaker' (Burke, quoted in Gusfield 1989: 34).

If we parents do not resist story that situates our disabled children as 'patients', we assign each child to 'a place in a moral order that subordinates him [or her] as an individual' (Frank 1997: 93). Might it be possible to change story – from the 'tragic, paranoic, or cataclysmic' (Randall 1995: 323) to a nar-rative that focuses less on bodily markers than on emancipatory gains for all differently embodied Others? With more awareness of intra-group discourse and of the linguistic magic of the dominant culture, the disability story might have an impact on social change. A 1990 study of the oral narratives of persons with disabilities demonstrates that by situating the disability culture as social minority, rather than as 'deviant', and by networking with other families with disabilities, there are 'transformational and liberating effects on . . . self-images', which may translate to more positive inscriptions conferred by the public (Phillips 1990: 855). Through cyberspace, perhaps, a broadcast medium with some 100 million voices and readers (Markel 1996: 119), the previously silenced or un-storied Other may achieve 'a new sense of identity as a communicator' (Johnson-Eilola 1994: 197). Virtual story has significant potential, not only for self-empowerment, but also as an engine of social change. But our 'highest goal', as Annette Kolodny argues, should be to make shifts in 'the images and *narrative structures* through which we compose the stories of our lives, [so that we may] alter the very experiences of those lives as well' (quoted in Hinchman and Hinchman 1997: 122, italics added).

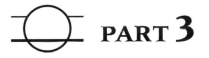 **PART 3**

# CULTURAL DISCOURSES

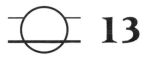 **13**

# Studying disability rhetorically

## Brenda Jo Brueggemann and James A. Fredal

### Introduction

Rhetoric is no stranger to disability; and disability is intimate, albeit anxiously, with rhetoric. In this chapter, we wish to illustrate that premise as we elaborate on some of the ways that rhetoric might add both depth and breadth to disability studies. We will focus on key moments or conventions in rhetoric's three largest sub-fields:

- the history of rhetoric,
- rhetorical theory, and
- rhetorical criticism,

and illustrate some of the generative ways rhetoric can explain, question, critique, and theorize disability from within those three areas.

### Rhetoric's history and disability

Throughout its 2500-year history, rhetoric has never been particularly friendly to 'disabled', 'deformed', 'deaf' or 'mute' people, the 'less-than-perfect' in voice, expression or stance. In fact, until fairly recently one could, without much injustice, define rhetoric as the cultivation and perfection of performative, expressive control over oneself and others. Though rhetorical theory has always devoted much, perhaps most, of its attention to the purely conceptual activities of inventing and arranging the 'available means of persuasion', it can never completely lose sight of the oral, performative communication of these means. Thus, in addition to the categories of 'invention', 'arrangement' and 'style' – steps in the composing of a speech – was the category of 'delivery', which defined not only proper pronunciation and accent, but gesture, facial expression and general bodily deportment as well. And while rhetoricians – those who elaborated theories of persuasive speaking – almost never afforded the canon of delivery, or *actio*, the same attention as they did *inventio* (invention), many orators – those who spoke in the assembly, the courts or for ceremonial occasions – were willing to admit that the performance of a speech was the most important aspect of the art of persuasive speaking. The orator Demosthenes, one of the most famous of the 'Attic' orators, for example, called delivery the first, second and third most important components of eloquence, a pronouncement which Cicero upheld (*De Oratore*, III. lvi. 213; Quintilian, *Institutes of Oratory*, XI. iii. 6–9). The persuasive power of a well-conceived and composed oration could be lost with a poor delivery, while, on the contrary, an effective delivery could overcome many faults in a composition.

While the particular principles, rules and proscriptions that make up the art of rhetoric vary from one age to the next, rhetoricians and orators took for granted that anyone who hoped to control the will of an audience had first to control their own voice and body. Most important to the delivery of a speech was the energy and propriety of the orator's performance: it must convey the force of the speaker's passionate conviction without transgressing cultural codes of conduct and deportment. If for Aristotle deformities or infirmities warranted a well-deserved death by exposure or 'euthanasia', it was much more the case that orators must be well formed and not only fully but perfectly functioning (Quintilian, *Institutes of Oratory*, XI. iii. 12–13). At rhetoric's height in pre-Macedonian Greece and, later, in the Roman republic, the *orator perfectus* who led the nation by virtue of his publicly performed orations had to embody all the classical public virtues, including energy, wilful self-control, and physical, intellectual and financial resourcefulness. Demosthenes, for example, was routinely upheld as an example of human virtue overcoming natural infirmity. He was, it seems, born with a weak and stuttering voice (Plutarch, *Lives of the Ten Orators*, 844 E–F). So shamed was he after his first oration that he shaved half of his head to prevent his going out in public while he practised his delivery. His practice of declaiming with pebbles in his mouth, or over the roar of pounding ocean surf – to overcome his natural speaking defects and to gain a more naturally powerful delivery – is one of the most well-rehearsed anecdotes in rhetorical history. Certainly it might also stand as an early example of rehabilitative 'technologies'.

For the next 2000 years, rhetoric has periodically added to, remodelled, or refurbished this classical model – the perfectly formed and fully franchised public representative – without substantially altering its foundations or structural supports. Roman rhetoric largely looked to and adopted from its Greek antecedents; but even in the act of borrowing, it also denounced them. Greek orators were upheld as models not only of excellent speaking, but of excellent public action. Demosthenes became the paragon of the civic leader of the *res publica*: a public-minded citizen capable of uniting, and thereby constituting, a community behind him. This was the model for Cicero as well as for Hume; for Quintilian – an educator and rhetorician in the late Roman

Empire – as well as for Thomas Jefferson (see, for example, Fliegelman 1993; Potkay 1994). More recently, the repeated layerings of new technologies of communication – from print to the telephone and television to the Internet – have shaped and reshaped traditional rhetorical principles, introducing new themes (such as 'secondary orality') even as traditional themes are fundamentally changed or forgotten (like the once vital canon of memory). How these technologies enable or disable rhetorical interactions, and for whom, is a question more complex and needing more specificity of focus than broad generalities like 'literacy' or 'electronic' can offer.

But throughout its history, rhetoric has, paradoxically, *itself* been denounced as a disabling pursuit. To the degree that persuasion was worked on auditors through such non-rational avenues as stylistic figures, alliterative diction or emphatic gestures, it crippled men's (audiences as well as speakers were routinely understood to be exclusively male) ability to deliberate coolly and rationally for themselves or to follow the truth. For philosophers like Plato as well as Christian apologists like St Jerome, arts of persuasion were suspect for their ability to lead people away from the revealed truths of religion or the discovered truths of dialectic. Though rhetoric required perfectly functioning bodies, its detractors also condemned it for appealing to the body and the senses at all: rhetoric used and relied upon the audience's common – that is, 'normal' – senses, emotions and passions to attain its goals. But even a perfectly feeling body could be deemed irrelevant to pure philosophy or revealed religion. And when the pursuit of truth did admit of rhetoric's usefulness, perfect bodies were again invoked as the conditions upon which this use could be employed. Thus while St Augustine championed classical rhetoric as useful to the conversion and edification of the faithful, their perfect hearing was essential to their being accepted into the faith (*On Christian Doctrine*). And while Plato eventually accepts rhetoric as a 'hand-maiden' to philosophy, he illustrates their difference through an ableist allegory of two horses pulling the chariot of the soul: one horse is perfect in form and loves the light, the other is 'crooked, heavy, ill put together . . . his color dark . . . is shaggy eared and deaf, hardly obedient to whips and spurs' (*Phaedrus*, 253 E).

Bodily deformity thus at once prevented any rhetorical achievement, while at the same time it symbolized the problem with rhetoric as a deceptive and sensuous art. When the canon of delivery received renewed attention in the elocution movement (roughly 1700–1900), this relationship went largely unchanged. Elocutionists (and rhetoricians in general) maintained the natural and immediate transmission of thoughts, feelings and beliefs through the stance, gestures, facial expressions and vocal qualities of the performer. That Black people could not blush signalled an absence of shame; that 'cripples' could not enact or voice their passions similarly signalled some inner spiritual or psychic lack. So pervasive was this Enlightenment fetish for bodily, performative signs of inner states that we currently use elocutionary terms to indicate characteristics of selfhood and personal agency: 'voice', 'stance', 'position', and 'posture'. Rhetoricians (for example, John Bulwer,

Juan Luis Vives) frequently either borrowed (stole) from deaf communities their gestural and expressive vocabularies for a hearing clientele and reader-ship, or ignored or condemned sign and gesture in favor of rhetoric's most highly prized resource: fluent speech (Alexander Bell, James Rush). The long struggle of deaf activists against oralist education and therapy has its roots, historically, in rhetoric's elocutionary movement. In sum, the historical relationship between rhetoric and disability has been neither peaceful or productive.

## Rhetorical theory

Given disability's troubled position within the history of rhetoric, the ques-tion might become: why even bother to take a rhetorical approach to dis-ability studies, to bring disability into rhetoric and rhetoric into disability? We think the answers lie in excavating rhetorical theory and rhetorical criti-cism, for what they are worth, in relation to disability. And in such excavating we would hope to rewrite not only the history, but possibly the present and future, of disability's place in rhetorical history. We would turn first to terms, the very bones of rhetorical theory. When we teach courses in rhetoric, or when we help graduate students prepare for Master's or PhD exams in rhetoric, we find ourselves – for better or worse – with a list of 'master' terms in hand. A recent list generated in a graduate seminar on the history of rhetoric included, for example: invention; arrangement; style; memory; delivery; ethos, pathos, logos; kairos; commonplaces; enthymeme; taste; sub-limity; tropes; proofs – artistic and non-artistic; metaphor; reason; language as: social behaviour, intention, interpretation, determining meaning, cre-ating knowledge, ideology, power; persuasion; argument; discourse; discur-sive formations; ethics; practical reasoning; speech acts; identification; consubstantiation; semiotics; pragmatics; 'grammar'; episteme (and epis-temic); dialogue; dialectic; deconstruction; 'literary' vs. 'ordinary'; belles let-tres; sermonic; Burke's pentad – act, scene, agent, agency, purpose; the rhetorical triangle – speaker, subject, audience; presence.

Were the challenge ever made, we are sure we could exhaust ourselves by locating the relevance of each of these terms in theorizing disability. But here we want to illustrate the potential power of rhetorical theory in disability studies by focusing on a few of these key terms.

### Persuasion

Like any discipline, rhetoric begins with defining itself. And in its beginning, in the first cited definition for rhetoric given by Corax and Tisias in 467 BCE, *persuasion* figures prominently: 'Rhetoric is the artificer of persuasion', they state simply. A hundred years later, in 350 BCE, Aristotle hands us what has become the 'standard' definition for rhetoric and he further aligns it with persuasion: 'Let rhetoric be [defined as] an ability, in each [particular] case, to see the available means of persuasion' (*Art of Rhetoric*, I. 1355a). Cicero (106–43 BCE), reputedly the greatest of the Roman (if not all) orators, echoes: rhetoric is 'the art of effective persuasion' (*De Oratore*). And although during the next 2500 years rhetoric often discarded 'persuasion' in favour of other more inclusive or more specific terms (rhetoric, like most disciplines, engages energetically in reinventing the wheel), the alliance between rhetoric and 'persuasion' remained strong. In the twentieth century, our principal rhetoricians still imply persuasion as they name rhetoric with phrases like 'to form attitudes or to induce actions' (Burke 1969: 46) or 'gaining the adherence of minds' (Perelman and Olbrechts-Tyteca 1969: 13).

To study the persuasion surrounding the construction and maintenance of disability – medically, aesthetically, linguistically, socially, economically, sexually (to name but a few) – would certainly be a fruitful endeavour. Questions we might begin with, generated by rhetorical definitions such as those offered above, include: who are the 'artificers' of disability? And how do they become so? What are all the *available* means of persuasion' when disability is argued about? How do those differ from the *existing* means or the *effective* means? How is persuasion used to 'form attitudes' or 'induce actions' or 'gain the adherence of minds' concerning disability?

When rhetoricians study persuasion and attempt to answer questions like these they often turn a more specific, microscopic lens onto certain other terms and configurations of rhetoric in order to help them then draw the bigger persuasive picture. They look (for example using Aristotle as their guide) at the three classical appeals (*pisteis*): *logos*, or the logic of the argument; *pathos*, or the passions of the audience; and *ethos*, the character of the speaker. How (and why, when and where) is the argument 'logically' made (*logos*)? Who are the audience of disability discourses, and how are they appealed to 'emotionally' (*pathos*)? How does the character of the speaker or writer get 'built' and 'delivered' (*ethos*)? To carry out the equation with disability in place: how (and why, when, and where) is a construction of disability established as logical? How is disability emotionally presented? (Why are its emotional tropes so limited to pity, depravation, degradation, inspiration and the like? What weight do these presentations carry in our culture?) And finally, what of the character of the disabled person – or of those who persuade about disability, whether disabled or not? How does their *ethos* contribute to the persuasive endeavour? (We might consider, as but one case, the arguments about *who* can do disability studies in the first place – see Oliver's chapter, this volume.)

### Commonplaces

We might also consider the 'commonplaces' of arguments surrounding disability. In classical rhetorical theory, 'commonplaces' were the standard sources for invention, the places (in the mind) one went to in order to discover (or invent) persuasive appeals. In Aristotelian rhetoric, the 'commonplaces' are, in essence, 'brainstorming' – where one begins looking in order 'to see [all] the *available* means of persuasion' (italics added). Establishing the greater and the lesser of the thing is often cited as the most foundational of the commonplaces. 'Which is the greater and lesser of disabilities? When is a disability greater or lesser?' These familiar questions are examples of the 'commonplace' arguments surrounding disability, perpetrators of persuasion about disability. And there are at least 28 more of these kinds of commonplaces in Aristotle's *Rhetoric* alone. Certainly, it might prove exhaustive and merely a 'mental exercise' to examine all 28 of these inventional commonplaces when disability is argued about. But we also think that such an exercise would begin to take us more broadly and deeply than some of our current limited ventures in disability studies. Such rhetorical studies of disability might have us looking, for example, at more than only medical models, or socio-political ones, or rehabilitative ones, or aesthetic ones; instead they might help us to look at what commonplaces undergird all of these models. And this, we think, would be theory-building at a new level.

## Rhetorical criticism

Currently, most activity in rhetoric is not in the area of theory-building, or even in speechifying, but in the criticism of cultural, ideological, political or aesthetic discourses. Nor is this criticism restricted to spoken or even written discourse. Current rhetorical critics examine gender portrayal on television, the appeal of family photographs, the actions of anti-nuclear activists or the discursive construction of sports personalities (Foss 1996). Rhetorical terms like those outlined above are used to analyse the ways in which meaningful activity shapes our thoughts, our bodies and our lives. For example, a rhetorical critic might examine how manufacturers of prosthetic devices establish their credibility (*ethos*) and appeal to the emotions (*pathos*) of a consuming audience, while explaining what their product does and how it works (*logos*). Thus, cochlear prostheses (implants) originally marketed to implant users failed to produce the demand that the manufacturer (the Cochlear Corporation) hoped for. A rhetorical analysis might explore how the Cochlear Corporation reconceived their appeal to address an audience of (parental) purchasers rather than of actual users, and how this shift necessitated an alteration in their logical and ethical appeals as well (like enlisting FDA approval for its use on children).

Other rhetorical critics, like Walter Fisher, working from the assumption that human understanding works primarily through the coherence and fidelity of stories, examine cultural practices and events as narratives (Fisher 1987). One might thus examine narratives of disabled persons (Quasimodo in *The Hunchback of Notre Dame* or the life of Bob Dole) or examine constructions of disability as narratives in and of themselves. Thus, any category of disability might be seen as a cultural story that is compelled to follow a familiar and appealing plot with predictable characters: the cripple, misfit or freak (rendered, as suggested above, along a few basic lines: pitiful victim, vicious savage, overcompensated savant, or gutsy overachiever), the potential (possibly platonic) love interest (consummated to the degree that the disability is overcome, compensated for or remedied), the philanthropic agent of change (the kind doctor, the long-suffering attendant, the disabled person him or herself, the federal government), the evil villain (the disability or the disabled person him or herself, or the cause of the accident, or the deadly disease-producing germ). In this critical, *rhetorical* light, Rudolph the Red-nosed Reindeer works as a misfit-becomes-leader disability narrative that appeals (a traditional term within rhetoric) to children and adults for specific reasons, satisfying culturally specific fears, hopes and desires, as all stories do. Rhetorical critics can read scientific, literary, legal or journalistic texts as stories – allegories about how a culture creates and enforces roles for its members, and the plots according to which those roles are expected to act.

These methods of rhetorical criticism work alongside a number of others currently in use: metaphorical criticism; pentadic (Burkean) criticism; fantasy-theme criticism; feminist, anti-racist, or queer criticism. In general, rhetorical criticism is moving away from attention to the 'great speaker, great speech' model, and towards larger, more complex and diffuse social movements, cultural trends and ideological power relations. Rhetorical critics understand theorists like Michel Foucault, Mikhail Bakhtin, Henry Louis Gates Jnr and Helene Cixous to be rhetorical theorists and critics because of the ways in which they reconceive the power of discourse to shape human thought and action. Rather than 'rhetorical criticism', *critical rhetoric* is becoming an increasingly popular term to describe the interest of rhetoricians in calling attention to and advocating changes in existing power imbalances and the 'discursive regimes' that maintain them. In this form, then, rhetoric as a theory, a practice and a tool for analysis is well aligned with the current direction of disability studies. Despite its inauspicious beginning, we are certain that rhetoric's long history and extensive vocabulary of textual strategies and tactics offers an unparalleled resource for analysing, understanding, and rethinking the nature of ability and disability, 'normal' and 'cripple'.

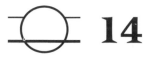 **14**

# Modern slogan, ancient script: impairment and disability in the Chinese language

## Emma Stone

> *Canfei*: (adj., pronounced tsan-fay) people with impairments: a common and derogatory Chinese term, translate as 'useless' or 'worthless'.
>    *Canji*: (adj., pronounced tsan-jee) people with impairments: an apparently new and neutral term, translate as 'disabled'.

### Setting the scene

Saturday, 16 March 1996. Beijing. The tape recorder is still running and we have been talking for over an hour. Hot water is added to the tea and Mr Liu's wife invites me to have more fruit. Mr Liu, a disabled artist and activist, continues:

> There are so many differences with the past. Before the 1980s, all the newspapers and broadcasts would call us *canfei* people. The word itself tells you so much! Under appeal from many disabled people, newspapers and the rest of the media changed and started using *canji* people. Since then, step by step, the rest of society has started to change.
>                       (field interview with Mr Liu, 16 March 1996)

The switch from the discouraged (because derogatory) term *canfei* to the apparently new and neutral term *canji* has been encapsulated in a Chinese government slogan, *canji erbu canfei*: 'disabled but not useless'. The slogan was coined and spread in the 1980s and, as is often the case with Chinese slogans, has gained relatively common currency. During nine months of fieldwork on disability and development in China, I came across the slogan frequently in conversation, in the press and on television, in both rural and urban areas of the Chinese mainland.

Of course, slogans (as with any spin-doctored soundbites) are notoriously suspect, particularly when promulgated by an undemocratic, quasi-

Communist, tank-despatching government. But is that sufficient grounds for dismissing the slogan as meaningless? The slogan is aimed at changing personal and public perceptions of disability. It is a direct attack on the more established aphorism, *canfei wuyong*: 'disabled person, good for nothing' which sums up the all-too prevalent hostility and disregard for disabled people in China. In contrast, 'disabled but not useless' appears closer to Western axioms which focus attention on abilities, not disabilities.

From my standpoint as a British postgraduate research student, the Chinese government's attempt to challenge disabling language and redefine disability seemed more in tune with Western disabled people's movements than with stereotypical representations of post-Mao China. Thus I found the slogan intriguing, even perplexing. Where had the preferred term, *canji*, originated? Was it new and neutral? These questions prompted me, after years of learning classical and modern Chinese, to think about the Chinese language in a new way. I began to interrogate the ancient Chinese script in search of clues to the meaning of impairment and construction of disability in a Chinese socio-cultural framework – in search also of a historical context within which to situate the decidedly modern-sounding slogan, *canji erbu canfei*.

The results of that search are summarized below with regard to

- the language of impairment and what this reveals about dominant Chinese perceptions of people with impairments;
- the language of 'normalcy' and 'non-normalcy' and the light this sheds on the construction of disability in China.

First, however, it is helpful to review the salient characteristics of the Chinese writing system.

## Ancient script

The written word has held, and continues to hold, a privileged position in Chinese history, politics, culture and society. A unified writing system has been in place since the first unification of the Chinese empire at the end of the third century BC and has served as 'one of the most effective instruments of political unification' (Gernet 1988: 32). In a vast empire marked by diversity of dialect, geography, custom and climate, the unified script enabled a remarkable degree of cultural conformity, centralized administration and imperial control. Moreover, Chinese characters or ideograms have long been invested with symbolic, even mystical, significance (Smith 1983). In short, the rich symbolism inherent in this ancient and enduring script offers fertile ground for language and culture analysis.

Every character corresponds to a semantic unit. Characters can be extremely complicated, containing many components. Each character has at least one Radical or dominant component which assists the grouping of characters in a dictionary and often imparts meaning. Additional meaning and sound are provided by other components in the character. There are 214 Radicals, the most complex of which requires 17 brush strokes. An individual character, including its Radical, may comprise as many as 37 brush strokes.

Many Chinese characters are symbols or stylized pictures and they can therefore provide important clues to socio-cultural perceptions and elite attitudes (Smith 1983). For example: the character for 'woman' comprises the symbol for a pregnant woman, thereby conveying the role of woman as child-bearer and the place of woman at home; in telling contrast, 'man' comprises the symbol for physical strength and a stylized picture of a field (see Figure 14.1). Anyone with a basic knowledge of gender issues in China's past and present will immediately make the relevant connections. Guisso (1981) has taken the project even further in his study of perceptions of women in classical texts and early Chinese script.

男 = 田 + 力

man = field + strength

女

woman = stylized picture of a pregnant woman

*Figure 14.1*

In the earliest Chinese lexicon (containing 9353 characters), Guisso identified 245 characters with the Woman Radical, of which 36 were descriptive. Of those, 28 pertained to temperament; over three-quarters were negative (e.g. lazy, jealous, garrulous), while the small number which might be described as positive still conformed to a Confucian world view which placed women in a strictly subordinate position to men.

The Guisso example is a convincing one. Nevertheless, deep-reading any written language is replete with pitfalls, particularly when the reader is an outsider and the script is ancient. Languages, like societies and cultures, constantly expand and change, and yet it would be churlish to ignore the insights offered by Chinese characters.

The findings outlined below are based on a recent analysis of Chinese characters and aphorisms (metaphors, proverbs, phrases), since these have occupied a significant place in Chinese oral and written culture. The main sources used are dictionaries of classical Chinese (Mathews 1943; Karlgren 1972), collections of popular phrases (Williams 1920; Huang 1964; Lip 1984; Yong 1996), and field notes taken in 1995 and 1996. Throughout this paper, passing reference is made to dominant Chinese cultural concepts and world views (especially those associated with Taoism and Confucianism, which are the most enduring and influential of Chinese philosophies) and conceptualizations of the bodymind and the individual (see Chan 1963; Lau 1979, 1988 for further information on Chinese philosophies; Kleinman 1980 and Kleinman *et al.* 1995 on Chinese conceptualizations of bodymind; Jenner 1994 and King and Bond 1985 on Chinese views of the individual, family and social relations *inter alia*).

## The language of impairment

*Canfei*, the term currently targeted for extinction, is a good starting point. The character *can* is grouped under the Bone-fragment Radical which carries strong connotations of death and destruction. Depending on context, *can* means damage, oppression and that which remains following destruction – the dregs. It is used to describe the setting sun, the waning moon, a dying breath, dying flowers, fallen women, broken vessels. *Fei* contains the meaning component 'to expel', hence it is used for 'to do away with', 'to get rid of', 'waste', 'useless', 'decrepit'. The combination of characters does not require further elucidation.

*Canfei* is certainly not the only term used to denote impairments. A careful search in the Karlgren (1972) and Mathews's (1943) dictionaries came up with over 150 individual impairment-specific characters used in Chinese texts, about 30 of which are still used in everyday speaking and writing. The dominant impairments or bodymind variations referred to are physical (especially lameness, short stature and hunched backs), visual, speech, hearing, and impairments which would nowadays be termed learning difficulties and mental health disorders but which, for the purpose of this analysis, are better translated as 'idiocy' and 'insanity' to distinguish them from more recent and outsider-influenced terminology. A good proportion of the 150 characters are descriptive, often denoting physical appearance, behaviour or manner of movement. Unsurprisingly, Radicals for Eye, Ear, Mouth, Foot, Walk, Lame and Mind or Heart occur frequently in impairment-specific characters, sometimes with added meaning from secondary components (see Table 14.1: *mang, xia, miao*).

Causation is identifiable in numerous impairment-related characters and is most visible in terms for penal mutilation, thus 'cut-off ear', 'cut-off foot' and 'cut-off nose' all feature the Knife component. Such specificity strongly suggests that perceptions of an individual with impairment vary/ied according to causation. The final example in Table 14.1, *gu*, 'insane', may also denote causation, since drinking poisonous worms was believed to induce insanity.

Several of the examples in Table 14.1 are grouped under the Sickness Radical and derive their meaning from the conjunction of the Sickness Radical with a component signifying the 'desired' state, thereby constructing a polarity of 'normative' and 'non-normative' (a point to which we shall return

*Table 14.1*    The language of impairment: descriptive and causation-specific characters

| Character | Radical | Component | Translation |
|-----------|---------|-----------|-------------|
| mang | Eye | die, destroy | blind |
| xia | Eye | damage, harm | blind |
| miao | Eye | small | one-eyed, low vision |
| lou | Person, man | crooked | hunched back |
| yu | Person, man | hillock, mound | hunched back |
| er | Ear | knife | cut-off ear |
| chi | Sickness | knowledge | idiot, stupid |
| dian | Sickness | true, real | insane |
| xian | Sickness | leisure | fits, epilepsy |
| que | Sickness | add + flesh | lame, crippled |
| long | Sickness | abundant | decrepit, deformed |
| yin | Sickness | sound | mute |
| gu | Worms | vessel | insane |

subsequently). At this stage, it is worth underlining the marked *absence* of divisions between illness and impairment in Chinese cosmobiological conceptualizations of the bodymind. Both impairments and illnesses are construed as products or signs of imbalance: internal imbalances of *yin* and *yang*, heat and cold; external imbalances in family and social relations, between ancestors and descendants, spirits and mortals, rulers and subjects. In Chinese cosmologies, where Cartesian dualisms of body versus mind do not rule as they do in the West, the bodymind is perceived as a microcosm of family, lineage, society, state, nature and cosmos. Therefore, imbalance in the bodymind might be attributed to a wide range of factors and blame is not necessarily attached to the individual or even to close family members. However, and crucially, this does not reduce the extent to which imbalance is cast as negative and undesirable, since imbalance is – by Chinese cosmological definition – a symbol of disorder, of departure from the ideal Way or the *Tao*. The use of the Sickness Radical, then, signifies the perception of impairment (and any bodymind imbalance) as noteworthy and undesirable because 'non-normative' and dis-ordering.

To return to the language of impairment, several characters contain clues which go beyond description, causation or naming as non-normative. References to poverty feature in many characters and aphorisms. Both *jian* (defect) and *jian* (lame) include a meaning component which denotes bitter cold and extreme hardship, while the proverbs 'poverty and illness – closely linked', 'poverty and hardship, much illness/impairment' and 'meet with impairment, poverty is inevitable' compound the associations (both cause and effect) of poverty and impairment. These characters and sayings convey more than the mere fact of the likely economic exclusion of people with impairments or the realities of poverty ratchets whereby poorer households are more prone to illness and impairment. In Chinese society and culture, poverty is feared and often despised: those who live in poverty are denoted by terms which frequently operate as terms of abuse. So, Beijing-dwellers mock *nongmin*: peasants, poor, poorly educated and unsightly; for much the same reason, Shanghai-dwellers use 'Jiangbei people' or 'Jiangbei swine' in name-calling (Honig 1989).

Impairment-related characters which double as terms of abuse are prevalent In their very composition, they speak volumes about negative perceptions of people with impairment. Many characters, mostly referring to 'idiots', 'simpletons' or 'mad people', are framed by Animal Radicals or contain components which denote devils or inanimate objects (see Table 14.2). Some of these, it may be argued, merely convey appearance (terms for hunched back), behaviour (correspondence between madness and rabies), or causation (madness-inducing worms or spirit-caused impairment).

Yet the frequency with which impairment words are used as abusive terms in everyday discourse in the 1990s and the findings of recent research on Chinese discourses of race (Dikotter 1992) and native place identity (Honig 1989) suggest that animal, devil and object associations carry deeper and more disturbing significance. Given the low place of animals in the Confucian world view, and the liminal and threatening position occupied by spirits and ghosts, it is highly probable that such characters communicate/d the diminished personhood of people and social groups with visible bodymind variations, whether those variations relate/d to physical or mental attributes, skin pigmentation, hair colour or speech patterns. The end result is the same: to dehumanize, to make Other.

The socio-cultural project of Otherness, in Chinese culture as in many Western cultures, is not limited to negative dehumanizing labels, as Barnes (1992), Shakespeare (1994) and Garland-Thomson (1997) have pointed out. Associations which appear positive, such as the ascription of special skills and virtues, also compound Otherness. In the Chinese script, virtues of

*Table 14.2* The language of impairment: dehumanizing characters

| Character | Component | Translation |
| --- | --- | --- |
| *yu* | monkey | stupid, idiot |
| *lu* | fish | stupid, idiot |
| *ai* | horse | stupid, idiot |
| *tao* | wood | stupid, blockhead |
| *dai* | wood | stupid |
| *chun* | worm | stupid |
| *kuang* | dog | insane |
| *ji* | dog | insane |
| *tuo-bei* | camel | hunchback |
| *tai-bei* | old horse | hunchback |
| *jian* | horse | deformed, defect |
| *hui* | devil or ghost | deformed |
| *chou* | devil or ghost | physical/moral deformity |

endurance and filial piety appear in many popular aphorisms, such as 'a lame tortoise walks a thousand miles', 'simple but loyal and filial', 'short stature, capable and alert' and 'a dwarf has many resources'. Similarly, the character *ru* means both 'dwarf' and 'literati' and *jiao* means both 'dwarf' and 'clever'. A common character for 'blind' (see Figure 14.2) comprises the symbols for Eye and Drum. It denotes a blind individual and, more specifically, a blind musician, thereby ascribing exceptional musical talent as compensation for visual impairment (an early example of this usage is found in the Confucian Classic, the *Book of Odes*, which dates to the pre-Christian era). However, proverbs and characters which appear positive are far outweighed by those which use impairment (especially visual impairment and inability to speak) as metaphors for ignorance, bewilderment, poor perception, futility, danger, falsity, suffering and exclusion. In the final analysis, projections of emotions and ascription of attributes, good or bad, all feed the self-same process of designating bodymind variation as a basis for different personhood.

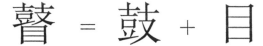

blind, blind musician = drum + eye

*Figure 14.2*

Aud Talle (1995: 71) has argued with respect to the Kenyan Maasai that to 'name the difference and mark it . . . indicates acceptance'. I argue that the same does not hold true with the Chinese language of impairment. Admittedly, a majority of characters convey appearance, manner or perceived notions of causation and might therefore be evaluated as neutral. However, the use of dehumanizing and Otherness-creating symbols to denote individuals with impairment must surely be taken as evidence of a cultural intolerance of impairment and bodymind variation. This argument is substantiated by further analysis of the Chinese language of 'normalcy' and 'non-normalcy'.

### The language of 'normalcy' and 'non-normalcy'

So far, analysis of the language of impairment has revealed a Chinese conceptualization of bodymind variation as undesirable, signifying departure from an ideal Way known as *Tao*, embodying Disorder (lack of *Tao*) in the realms of bodymind, family, society, nature and cosmos. Impairments are situated in opposition to *Tao* (Order) and thereby a polarity of impaired and non-impaired, normative and non-normative is created.

What is particularly fascinating about this process is that exacting notions of normalcy exist in a culture which is otherwise known for notions of complementarity rather than polarity, fluctuation rather than fixity. Many Westerners are aware, for example, of the complementary dualism enshrined in the Chinese Taoist concept of *yin* and *yang*: the idea that male and female (light and dark, heat and cold) complement each other and ideally coexist in a state of harmonious balance. Perhaps the point most often overlooked by Western outsiders is that harmony and hierarchy are not mutually exclusive concepts in Chinese cosmologies. As Robert Guisso points out in his study of the place of women in Chinese classical culture, harmony is viewed as wholly dependent on a fixed hierarchical order in which women are subordinate to men, youth is subordinate to age, subjects are subordinate to rulers (Guisso 1981). Similarly, while impairments and illnesses may be construed as signs of imbalance with potential for balance to be restored, they are equally signs of Disorder situated in direct opposition to ideals of *Tao*.

To illustrate the point further, it is worth exploring three conceptual characters: *quan*, *zheng* and *ding*. Each reveals what Nicolaisen (1995: 39) terms the 'cultural perception of the biological constitution of the human being itself' which, in China, is a fixed notion of a 'normative' bodymind.

*Quan* translates as complete, entire, whole. To be complete is to be perfect. Thus, when the *quan* character is framed by the Ox Radical, it denotes 'a bullock of all one colour, perfect in all its parts and fit for sacrifice'; when framed by the Sickness Radical, it means 'to cure' or 'restore to wholeness'. To be *bu quan* or *shi bu quan* is to be not complete, to be 'deformed'. *Zheng* denotes the orderly, proper, regular and orthodox. It encapsulates the essence of Confucianism as a philosophy which prizes orthodoxy and the middle way, leaving no room for excess, extreme or deviation. As regards the bodymind, any variation or difference is undesirable *because* it is unorthodox. Accordingly, the still common phrase *wu guan bu zheng* ('the five senses/organs/parts are not in their proper place, not orderly') is used for an individual with physical, sensory, behavioural impairments, facial disfigurement, scabies, leprosy and so on (Schak 1988). These two conceptual characters underwrite the perception that to have any form of bodymind difference is to be 'disorderly' and 'incomplete', hence heterodox and undesirable.

Where *quan* and *zheng* might be situated within cosmological or cosmobiological discourses, *ding* spans the cosmological and the everyday or public spheres. *Ding* is one of the 'Heavenly Stems'. More significantly, it is an administrative category which, throughout much of imperial Chinese history, denoted the taxable individual: able-bodied, able-minded, male and aged between 16 and 60 (Ho 1959; Twitchett 1970). The *ding* was the focus of population registration and liable to military and labour conscription, grain and monetary taxation. The character itself exudes the hegemony of dominant, able-bodied, male normalcy which marked public life in imperial China and the legacy of which is still very much apparent in the 1990s: *ding* is a picture of a nail – solid, strong, straight and useful (Figure 14.3).

丁

adult, able-bodied male; nail; heavenly stem

*Figure 14.3*

The classification of *ding* enshrined the 'normative' bodymind, taking normalcy out of the cosmological and embedding it in public discourse. What may have begun as a compassionate and helpful attempt to acknowledge economic hardship premised on impairment became an administrative, legislative and fiscal category which institutionalized the Otherness of people with impairments as diminished persons, while conveying and reinforcing the normative standard of the *ding*. This process was compounded by the categorization and subcategorization of those who were not *ding*: childless widows and widowers, orphans, the solitary (for, in China, little is more heterodox than being without family) and people with impairments – all of whom were classified as the *qiuling* or 'odds and ends'. They were set apart from and in opposition to the administrative norm. Within the 'odds and ends', specific categories were created for individuals with different degrees of impairments. Is it to imperial China that the ignominious award for earliest example of *disability* labels should be given?

Records of disability classifications date back at least as far as the legal and administrative statutes of the Tang dynasty which spanned the seventh to tenth centuries, and it is more than likely that the classifications were not new then, since innumerable facets of Tang administration owed their origins to the Han dynasty (206 BC–220 AD). The classifications are drawn from the *Hu Ling* or *Household Statutes* and are listed in full, albeit in a footnote, in Twitchett's text on financial administration in the Tang dynasty (1970: 212):

> All such persons as are blind in one eye, deaf in both ears, lacking two fingers on one hand or three toes from one foot, who have lost either their big toe or thumb, who are bald-headed and without hair, have a chronic discharge, dropsy or any large tumours, shall be considered partially disabled [*can ji*].
>
> Such persons as are idiots or dumb, dwarfed, with deformed spines, or lacking one limb, shall be considered seriously disabled [*fei ji*].
>
> Such persons as are completely insane, lacking two limbs, or blind in both eyes, shall be considered totally disabled [*du ji*].

The classifications were deployed in all facets of public life: in land allocation and financial administration, with regard to military and labour conscription, individual and family taxation (Ho 1959; Twitchett 1970) and also in imperial China's extensive legal codes, which made special allowances for disabled criminal offenders in the second and third grades of disability (Johnson 1979; Chiu 1980).

To summarize so far, the disability categories, whether by design or default, consolidated notions of different and diminished personhood based on impairment, constructing people with impairments in opposition to the administrative and cosmological norm of *ding*. Administrative in function, *ding* and the disability categories corresponded closely to cosmological concepts of complete and not-complete, orthodox and heterodox. Thus it makes sense to write about a language of disability as well as a language of impairment in the ancient Chinese script. Moreover, given that the lowest of the disability classifications is termed *canji*, we must conclude that *canji*, as a label for disabled people, is far from new. Nor can it be said to be neutral, since it carries the weight of centuries of administrative and cosmological demarcation between 'normative' and 'non-normative' bodyminds. With these findings in mind, we return briefly to the 1990s and the slogan which prompted inquiry.

## Modern slogan

Throughout the world the language of impairment and disability is changing. Increased international awareness of disability issues has resulted in a plethora of definitions and redefinitions, medical, social and political. Old words carry new meanings which have more to do with a global discourse of disability and rehabilitation than with indigenous cultural and historical concepts of bodymind variation. This process is illustrated in anthropological studies on Zaire, Borneo, Somalia, Kenya and Botswana which flag up the difficulties of translating the international (for which read Western) term 'disabled' into local languages (see Devlieger 1995; Helander 1995; Ingstad 1995; Nicolaisen 1995; Talle 1995 for case studies, Whyte 1995 and Miles 1996 for discussion). Often, words which originally denoted individuals with physical impairments are used as a unifying category for all individuals with impairments, thereby imposing outsider discourses with little consideration for indigenous conceptualizations.

In China too, new and global discourses are at work. Historical and linguistic research reveals age-old indigenous classifications of disability and socio-cultural conceptualizations of the bodymind which are particular to China, yet there appears to be a perceived need within China to coin a new term or give new meaning to an old term which will serve as a single umbrella category for all impairments and be an adequate translation for the Western term 'disabled'. The official definition now employed in mainland China divides the umbrella category, *canji*, into five subsets which conform to international agency definitions rather than indigenous perceptions or classifications. It is surely not surprising that the creation and promulgation of the slogan *canji erbu canfei* and the restructuring of official disability definitions followed so close upon China's re-entry into the international arena and the designation of 1982 to 1992 as the United Nations Decade of Disabled People. Nor is it any less surprising that the Chinese government's attempt to adopt internationally acceptable disability discourse has often exceeded, even dangerously, the coining of a new slogan (see the analysis of Chinese eugenics and disability legislation in Stone 1996).

Perhaps global or Westernizing discourses transposed to non-western contexts are no bad thing? After all, most Western diplomacy and reportage on China is preoccupied with winning the Chinese market and bringing the Chinese government round to international (Western) perceptions of human rights. In the final analysis, only time will tell whether the transplant of Western-evolved disability discourses into non-Western contexts works for or against the lives of individual disabled people.

## Conclusions

In this chapter, I have explored the ancient Chinese language of impairment with brief reference to cultural concepts and perceptions. In so doing, I have followed Whyte's recommendation that impairment (as distinct from disability) should be framed as a 'cultural and social issue, rather than a medical or technical one' (Whyte 1995: 285). I have also searched the Chinese script for language which goes beyond the communication of appearance, causation or behaviour . . . language which feeds into the construction of *disability*.

The research findings reveal that bodymind variation is significant in Chinese culture. Variation is cast in cosmological discourse as counter to the 'normative' bodymind. The fact that this occurs within a context which knows no bodymind dualism, sees the individual as a relational, family-centred and family-dependent being, and is otherwise known for a world view premised on complementarity and fluid balance, does little to soften the exacting notions of normalcy. These notions are nowhere more marked than in the three conceptual characters *quan, zheng* and *ding. Ding* in particular spans cosmological and public discourse, functioning as an administrative norm: those considered not *ding* were set apart and subdivided according to what may be the oldest disability labels in recorded history.

Chinese characters have clearly played their part in communicating and consolidating dominant perceptions of impairment and disability. Without doubt, they have much to reveal about indigenous and age-old conceptualizations. Such knowledge is vital if we are to begin to explore the articulation of new with older concepts, global with indigenous discourses.

Inevitably, the fear must be that new discourses imposed or imported may give an impression of newness, neutrality and positive change without fundamentally challenging or dismantling the cultural and material structures constituting disability in China. Slogans are empty words, surely? At this point, we might do well to revisit the scene set at the outset, rewind the tape and listen to Mr Liu's words more attentively.

> There are so many differences with the past. Before the 1980s, all the newspapers and broadcasts would call us *canfei* people. The word itself tells you so much! Under appeal from many disabled people, newspapers

and the rest of the media changed and started using *canji* people. Since then, step by step, the rest of society has started to change.

(Mr Liu, 16 March 1996)

In China, in the 1990s, there are people like Mr Liu for whom the slogan has great worth. If the slogan sounds a note of defiance, acts as a retort to those who mock and awakens others to the idea that discrimination is disabling, then it cannot be dismissed as mere propaganda.

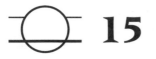 **15**

# Bodies, brains, behaviour:
# the return of the three stooges
# in learning disability

**Murray Simpson**

### Introduction

In recent years the learning disability field has been heading for fragmentation in terms of service philosophy. In the wake of normalization, critiques,
counter-critiques and alternative models, some people have shied away from
any encounters with theory and have adopted an intuitive empiricism. Alan
Tyne, for instance, suggests that 'the critiques [of normalization] have happened at some remove from the lives of people with disabilities' (Tyne 1992:
45). However, simply to ignore the theoretical dimension of learning disability would be naively to assume that 'what you can't see can't harm you'.
Others have tried to reassess the history of learning disability, perhaps in
order to identify pitfalls, lost opportunities, or to trace lines of determination.
Adopting an approach which uses discourse analysis, I want to argue that the
contemporary confrontation with history and theory is born out of the fact
that programmes based on older forms of power are running up against the
new technologies and models. Additionally, I want to suggest that for the past
200 years, the discourse on intellectual impairment has basically involved
the manipulation of three elements (intelligence, behaviour, and the organic
and functional impairment of the body). In addition, each 'revolution' and
mutation of the field (discursive, policy and practice) has been more or less
directly associated with the manoeuvring of these elements. Throughout this
chapter, I will use the term *learning disability* very deliberately, to describe a
field of policy, academic and professional discourse. In the context of any
study of discourse, substitution of terms is never likely to be satisfactory. In
line with the widely expressed view of *people with learning difficulties* themselves, I will use that term when specifically referring to people as opposed to
the nexus in which they may be caught.

It is important to make clear at the outset that I am not trying to suggest that these are the only significant elements involved in developments in theory or practice, or that there has ever been uniformity in the field. Neither would I wish to underplay the various modifications and mutations which all of the elements have undergone. The aim of this chapter is to demonstrate the close association between changes in discourse and changes in the way society responds to people with learning difficulties and, indeed, *constitutes* them as objects of knowledge and as subjects. I wish to take a number of concepts of learning disability, consider how each has deployed the three elements and explore the consequences of so doing. Most of the conceptual models relate roughly to different historical points, although they do not always divide neatly into discrete historical periods. The first model is primarily associated with the earliest phase of the development of a distinct discourse on 'idiocy', and is typified by the 'physiological method' of Edouard Seguin.

## Physiological treatment

Seguin's work is widely cited as marking a watershed in thinking about idiocy (e.g. Scheerenberger 1983; Trent 1995). Without wishing to go into more detail than is necessary here, Seguin's work involved an essentially pedagogical treatment of idiot children, based on muscular, sensory and intellectual training. Proponents of this approach claimed that the use of scientific methods of pedagogy could produce marked improvements in the levels of intellectual, physical and social functioning of idiot children. The work of Seguin and others spawned the first generation of institutions across Europe and North America. Some commentators have emphasized what they see as a 'psychological' orientation of this approach, with strong resonance with the growth and application of learning theory in the 1950s and 1960s (essentially on the basis of an optimism regarding change and development) (for example, Talbot 1964; Ryan and Thomas 1987). However, such interpretations miss the point somewhat inasmuch as psychology did not exist as an independent discipline at that time. Seguin operated in the field of medical psychology even before he completed his medical degree (and this perhaps leads to an altogether different interrogation of his work – specifically, how was it possible that a discourse of pedagogy could become deployed within a medical framework?).

Seguin's definition of idiocy (albeit not his first) was:

> *Idiocy is a specific infirmity of the cranio spinal axis, produced by deficiency of nutrition in utero and neo nati.* It incapacitates mostly the functions which give rise to the reflex, instinctive, and conscious phenomena of life; consequently, the idiot moves, feels, understands, wills, but imperfectly; does nothing, thinks of nothing, cares for nothing (extreme cases), he is a minor legally irresponsible; isolated, without associations; a soul shut up in imperfect organs, an innocent.
>
> (Seguin 1866: 39–40, author's italics)

Seguin adopts an organic aetiology and then, more significantly for what came next in his text, identifies idiocy as primarily a disorder of 'physiology', i.e. of the *functions* of the body, as opposed to the 'anatomy' or structures of the body. This is where some commentators become confused; Seguin's pedagogy was not so much about improving scholastic or *social* functioning of his idiot pupils. These were ultimate aims of course, but the direct objective of physiological treatment was to improve the functioning of the body and mind through stimulation and training. In other words, it targeted what had been made the definitive characteristics of idiocy. It wasn't about educating idiots in the sense of imparting knowledge and abilities so much as it was about ameliorating the idiocy itself.

## Pathological nosology

A later group of physicians began to explore the pathological aspects of idiocy in more detail. In particular, William Ireland constructed one of the first recognizably modern medical classifications of idiocy. In it, ten species of idiocy are identified: genetous, microcephalic, eclampsic, epileptic, hydrocephalic, paralytic, cretinism, traumatic, inflammatory, and idiocy by deprivation (Ireland 1877: 40–1). Building directly on the work of Seguin and his contemporaries (and at their injunction), these physicians used the newly formed institutional populations as experimental subjects. The objectives were: the identification of pathological causes; differential diagnosis and prognosis; and, where and when possible, interventions and cures specific to the different pathological types. With this discursive apparatus, the matter of social competence takes only a secondary position. However, Ireland did regard pathological classification as complimentary to psychic, that is, intelligence-based, ones. 'The human mind, bounded in its insight, requires to look at the subject in two aspects [mental and pathological] and for the same reason that we require to see a solid body on every side, unless it happens to be transparent' (Ireland 1877: 39).

## Psychology – intelligence testing

Once it was established as a discipline in its own right, the first major development in psychology relevant to the learning disability field was intelligence testing, initiated by Alfred Binet. IQ testing is slightly difficult to locate insofar as it has been associated with a number of quite different positions, though most particularly with eugenics. What is significant is that in IQ testing, questions of impairment of body or mind, or of behavioural competence, are bracketed (though IQ testing is compatible with the study of the other elements). The following is a typical example of classification based on IQ.

*Idiots* – were defined as persons with a mental age of not more than thirty-five months or, if a child, an IQ less than twenty-five.

*Imbeciles* – were defined as persons with a mental age of between thirty-six and eighty-three months, or, if a child, an IQ between twenty-five and forty-nine.

*Morons* – were defined as persons with a mental age between eighty-four and 143 months inclusive or, if a child, an IQ between fifty and seventy-four.

(American Association for the Study of the Feebleminded 1921, quoted in Race 1995: 17)

IQ testing is further complicated by the fact that Binet himself insisted on the mutability of IQ and did not believe that idiocy was an arrest of development, both of which were reversed by most of those who adopted and developed IQ testing. Binet argued that

The exact nature of this inferiority is not known; and today without other proof, one very prudently refuses to liken this state to that of an arrest of normal development. It certainly seems that the intelligence of these beings has undergone a certain arrest; but it does not follow that the disproportion between the degree of intelligence and the age is the only characteristic of their condition.

(Binet, no date [1916])

This suggests that Binet saw his role as very much complementary to medicine. The important issue here, then, is what the role played by IQ testing was in each instance of its use. How was it possible for such finely differentiated intellectual grading to appear and what effects were produced? The fundamental condition which made such refined classification possible was, again, the existence of the institutional populations. It was in such establishments in Paris that Binet was presented with the groups of sufficient size to compare and classify. Three main functions can be discerned: first, classifying institutional and school populations for 'appropriate' schooling; second, by extension, matching individuals to appropriate social positions and employment; and, third, to demonstrate the fixed nature of IQ and the causal association between low intelligence and a range of social vices (see, for example, Block and Dworkin 1976).

## Behavioural psychology

From around the 1950s a growing number of clinical psychologists, mainly working in or from institutions for mental defectives, began to experiment with the application of behavioural techniques of training and behaviour modification. Significant among this work was that of O'Connor and Tizard (1956), who attempted to demonstrate the effectiveness of behavioural pedagogy in 'turning out socially competent citizens' (p. 7), teaching mental defectives to perform basic manual work and become financially self-supporting. In parallel with these experiments, there was also a move towards conceptual modification of mental deficiency to a more behavioural orientation. Given the medical domination of the field at that time, it is unsurprising to find that elements of behaviour are moved into a more primary position in defining and diagnosing mental deficiency without organic impairment actually being removed. O'Connor and Tizard outline six components to mental deficiency: anatomical and physiological, intellectual, educational, social competence, occupational and temperamental/moral (p. 12).

Although not strictly a definition of mental deficiency, these components have strong resonance with a contemporaneous definition of mental deficiency from Doll as comprising:

(1) Social incompetence, due to
(2) low degree of intelligence as a result of
(3) incomplete development which is
(4) permanent,
(5) obtains at maturity and derives from
(6) constitutional hypoplasia, pathology or dysmetabolism.

(Doll 1948, quoted in Race 1995: 19)

Doll's definition is particularly significant in the way in which the social competence is given primacy, with intelligence having secondary position and organic impairment appearing only as the originating cause. Behavioural approaches necessarily *imply* other components in supplying primary causation, but they invariably relegate the significance of those components in relation to the presenting 'problem' of mental deficiency and, most importantly, what to do about it.

## Reassessing discursive change

In this chapter I have selected and sketched four conceptual models of idiocy, mental deficiency and retardation. These are clearly not the only four models which have existed and shaped societal responses and provisions for people with learning difficulties. However, each corresponds to certain 'discontinuities' in the nexus of learning disability over the past 170 years or so: the initial growth of the pedagogical asylum; the foundations of medical specialization and pathological differentiation; the rise of eugenics and custodialism; and the impetus towards deinstitutionalization and normalization. What conclusions can be drawn from such an analysis?

First, the discursive shifts described do not correspond to moves towards the deeper understanding of the 'truth' of learning disability. The behavioural model, for example, is not more correct than the medical model in downgrading the significance of pathological types and the aetiology of intellectual impairment, it is simply a repositioning of the elements in the discursive nexus. The 'truth' of learning disability was reconstituted much more than it was actually advanced. This is broadly true for all of the shifts described, notwithstanding any additional knowledge which may have been added in the period. Instead, the modifications of the constellation of elements have been essentially tactical and strategic, advancing alternative institutional practices and interests.

Second, these apparently simple and sometimes innocuous acts of repositioning have had very profound significance insofar as they have provided the conditions in which it has become possible to think and act in new ways. Often, perhaps invariably, the effects of these events have unfolded with little significance deriving from the intentions of those involved in the generation and regeneration of the discourse. For example, in constituting idiocy as a physiological, as opposed to anatomical, impairment, Seguin and the physiological educators were able to define their practices which improved the functioning of idiots as ameliorative actions on idiocy itself, even though they left the organic impairment untouched. This is unthinkable in a model centred on pathological anatomy. Paradoxically, the pedagogical asylums which developed, based on the physiological method, became laboratories in which the more scientific and differentiated pathological discourse developed, eventually surpassing the physiological as the discourse of the idiot asylum. As noted above, IQ testing arose on the basis of classifying and differentially treating the new asylum population. The fixity of both the pathological and intelligence testing discourses came, in turn, to fuel a resurgence of eugenics in the first quarter of the century despite the lack of such a connection in the initial discourse of either. In a further twist, the subsequent inversion of the relative positions of pathology and behaviour meant that the application of behavioural techniques constituted actions on mental deficiency, as opposed to merely actions on the mentally deficient. The fortunes of people with learning difficulties, it appears, have risen and fallen in line with pedagogical optimism.

As I indicated at the outset, these are not the only conditions necessary for the movements in the learning disability field to which I have alluded. Indeed, James Trent argues that the fundamental determinant of the conditions in which different concepts thrive or fail is the economy (Trent 1995). Undoubtedly there will be other factors, localized or general, which have come to provide the actual conditions in which these theoretical routes were opened, and each needs to be carefully explored in greater detail. However, as well as attempting to cause some level of disruption to at least this one dimension, my attempts to undermine the continuity provided by the basic discursive set cast doubt on some of the attempts to transcend the current theoretical blockages. There are a number of such candidates around: normalization, framework of accomplishments, quality of life, ordinary life, even the social model of disability. However, it is questionable as to whether these go deeply enough to actually provide sufficient explanation of how we have come to pose the questions we have and in the manner we have; how, for instance, we are constrained by discursive regimes to think in certain ways, and are given specific and limited theoretical options for change. This analysis leads to the implication that it cannot be assumed that simply giving choices and self-determination to people with learning difficulties neces-sarily allows for any meaningful redefinition of the scope of subjectivities, materially and discursively constructed, into which they are inserted. People's choices are conditioned and limited by forces which are not so easily perceived as we might think.

To approach the matter from a different angle, even though definitions of learning disability have changed many times and have always been contested and plural at any given moment, despite also the fact that there have been many, often quite radical, changes to services, there has been another deeper level of continuity over the past 200 years, which attention to superficial questions not only avoids, but actively conceals. That continuity is provided in the way in which competence and liberty are connected to one another, the underlying theme being that people with learning difficulties must demonstrate their competence prior to being granted autonomy. This is the direct inversion of the principle of social intervention which holds for the rest of us.

## Community care and learning disability

Identifying a single, or any, definition of learning disability associated with the broad rubric of community care is extremely difficult. It is perhaps char-acteristic of care in the community not to adopt any clear mechanism of its own for defining and identifying client group types (paradoxically, given its techno-bureaucratic orientation). As far as adults with learning difficulties are concerned, they are generally presented to social work agencies already assessed and defined as having a learning disability at a much younger age, most likely by psychologists working in educational or medical sectors. At the same time, however, it can fairly easily be discerned that at the discursive level care in the community does not easily accommodate issues of intelli-gence or medical pathology; they have no immediate relevance for the assessment for, or delivery of, services. Behavioural competence is certainly a crucial issue, though specifically related to 'independence' as the primary objective of services. Community care also introduces a number of radically new elements: consumer choice, markets, cost-efficiency and suchlike.

Also, care in the community is itself is a prime example of practices made possible by discursive innovation. Prior to 1979 there was a sharp division in government policy between the economic and social (Wilding 1992: 109). The language of social policy was such that, for all political sides, the user of services could not be construed as a 'consumer' in any coherent sense. The discourse of the economy simply did not apply. However, 'community' per-forms a neat discursive connection in being the physical and conceptual link point between individuals as consumers, taxpayers and as having 'care needs'. The community paid, the community used. By creating a policy around this new locus the discourse of the economy entered that of social policy (and arguably vice versa, though to a lesser extent).

Prefiguring care in the community, the principle of normalization opened up the possibility of linking competence enhancement (and by implication, 'incompetence management') in the same order and sequence, discursively speaking, as 'moral rights', 'dignity', 'social and personal relations'. Elements diverse and unconnected by origin became drawn together into a single (though internally diverse) strategy of knowledge and power. The elements formed not so much a sequence perhaps as a matrix into which elements are inserted, unified and directed. The behavioural orientation of normalization and its parallels was and remains strong. However, as Felce (1996) notes, the supplanting of normalization by a discourse of community care has led to a decline in emphasis on development and competence enhancement in services. Unlike Felce, however, I think this is an important opportunity to critically reappraise the competence–liberty connection.

It is noteworthy that, among the designated community care groups, issues of development, skills acquisition, etc. figure most strongly in relation to people with learning difficulties. The rise of the 'Individual Programme Plan' in the 1980s typifies the close equation of competence enhancement with service function and success. But there are at least two senses in which concepts of competence might be used without connecting it to liberty: first, as a direct desire, 'I want to learn car maintenance'; or, second, as a means to an end, 'I want a place of my own, so I need to learn how to . . .' Taking the liberty–competence link as self-evident and inevitable incurs certain other errors, for instance, of thinking that freedom necessarily comes with reduced professional presence, and that this in turn comes with increasing competence. For some this may be true, but for many it won't be, especially those with more severe learning difficulties or multiple impairments for whom high levels of support will always be a reality. It also assumes that there is nothing fundamentally wrong, or at least changeable, about the relations between people with learning difficulties and professionals because these are the inevitable result of the learning disability. Competence is not liberation, though it may form part of it for some individuals. Neither is the capacity to live independently 'progress' if that independence is accompanied by unemployment, squalor, and lack of meaningful relations.

Trent (1995) notes that the discourse on learning disability has become focused on the person. Person-centred approaches are justified on the basis of technocratic as well as ethical reasons; they permit resource targeting and needs-led provision. However, the danger of such an exclusive orientation to the discourse of community care is that it generally fails to recognize regimes of power and discourse, and to acknowledge that the main need of people with learning difficulties is for society to stop oppressing them. Even those developments widely recognized as having such anti-oppressive potential, such as self-advocacy, liberating research methods, user-involvement, can easily exist within the discursive framework described. For certain, they all came out of this dominant framework in one way or another. What person with learning difficulties, for instance, came up with the term 'self-advocacy'? If one has to invent a special name to describe what most people take for granted, then one ought to be immediately suspicious.

Choices and actions occur within spaces. On one dimension, these spaces are discursive. They are 'subjectivities' constructed by what is said and done, constituting what we 'are': people with learning difficulties, social workers, academics, parents, etc. Feeling and *being* free to determine one's actions within that space is all well and good, but it is somewhat fanciful to think that inattention to the forces which constitute that space means that one is free from constraint. The biggest constraint is often on what can be thought.

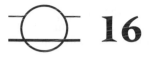 **16**

# Joseph F. Sullivan and the discourse of 'crippledom' in progressive America

**Brad Byrom**

At the age of 4, Joseph F. Sullivan contracted the polio virus. As he grew, his inability to use his legs, his limited arm function and his use of a wheelchair left little doubt in the minds of contemporaries that Sullivan would always be a 'cripple'. ('Cripples', according to most early-twentieth-century definitions, were individuals with physical impairments of one or more limbs.) In the late nineteenth-century American society in which Sullivan grew up, being crippled signified to most a dark and uncertain future excluded from such normal social relations as employment and marriage. Born to working-class parents in rural Arkansas, Sullivan's prospects did indeed seem bleak. His inability to walk made both education and employment unlikely prospects. In fact, Sullivan recalled, his own family could foresee only 'a life of utter uselessness and dependence' (Gray 1921: 11). Given such grim connotations it is of little surprise that Sullivan initially found being a cripple a source of great discomfort and pain. During his youth, Sullivan repeatedly felt the sting of a label that begrudged him a 'normal' childhood; he felt the discomfort of stares from both adults and children, and experienced the humiliation of being denied access to education. Reflecting on his childhood, Sullivan later wrote, 'almost everybody you met – yes, the grown ups especially – stared at you – blinked and rubbed their greedy eyes' (1921a: 3).

However, Sullivan did not spend his life mired in the obscurity of mendicancy. Due to his personal resilience and, more importantly, a bit of historical good fortune, Sullivan overcame the social and cultural barriers constructed by the non-disabled that prevent most disabled persons from attaining education and employment. Given only occasional access to public schooling throughout the first 16 years of his life, Sullivan struggled to gain the knowledge he so craved. Finally, at the age of 16 he used proceeds from newspaper sales to purchase a team of goats to help with transportation. The goats provided the mobility Sullivan needed to formalize his education. Upon high school graduation, however, Sullivan once again met a barrier – this time a barrier to employment. Sullivan sought a job with the local newspaper in Imboden, Arkansas, but was denied an opportunity on the basis that he could not climb the stairs to the newspaper's offices. Sullivan cleverly proved his ability to overcome the barrier, however, by climbing into the building through a rear window. Soon after acquiring editorship of the paper, Sullivan launched a successful campaign to become mayor of Imboden. In winning election before his twenty-first birthday, it was claimed, Sullivan became the youngest mayor ever in the United States (Gray 1921). Eventually, he married and settled into a life as an educator and an advocate for crippled children. His life work became that of establishing educational opportunities for all crippled children, an effort which gained momentum during the progressive era and in which his became a leading voice.

The importance of Sullivan's story as it relates to the evolution of disability discourse lies in its demonstration of the connections between life experience, the broad social discourses which exist at any point in history, and the evolution of disability discourse. Sullivan's initial inability to gain access to education, followed by the success he experienced upon graduating from high school, encouraged him to work for the establishment of educational opportunities for all crippled children. Yet his goals would likely have failed to gain an audience had they not meshed with a larger *progressive* discourse centring on themes of efficiency and science. This broad social discourse profoundly affected the definitions of disability created by Sullivan and other members of his reform-minded generation. Themes of efficiency first pushed along Sullivan's educational agenda, before the progressive faith in science overwhelmed his goals in ways he could scarcely comprehend. (For a discussion of the role of efficacy and the importance of science in progressive reform, see Haber 1964; Wiebe 1967.)

By the standards of early-twentieth-century disability discourse, Sullivan's achievements provided him with the rhetorical right to reject the label of 'cripple'. During both the progressive era and the years of American involvement in World War I (1890–1919), numerous writers reasoned that an individual gainfully employed should no longer be considered a cripple (Blake 1917; Dowling 1917, 1918; Avis 1918). Given the centuries-old association between cripples and begging, a tradition codified in the United States and abroad by laws protecting the cripple's right to beg, it is not surprising that individuals with physical impairments who found work came to be considered something more than 'cripples'. In both London and New York, for instance, cripples received exemptions from vagrancy laws restricting public begging (Ringenbach 1973). Such individuals, whom contemporaries imagined had overcome their physical impairments, exceeded the traditional bounds of what Sullivan referred to as 'crippledom'. In doing so, they gained a degree of respect not traditionally afforded individuals with physical disabilities. Such cripples received a remarkable amount of press during the war years. While stories concerning successful cripples had been popular for some time, the prospect of thousands of disabled veterans returning from the battlefields of Europe thrust the life stories of Sullivan and others into the national spotlight during and immediately after World War I. As one of the most highly publicized of such individuals, Sullivan faced a seemingly diffi cult choice – to distinguish himself from other cripples or to accept the label of cripple and identify with his less fortunate 'brothers'.

In the literature Sullivan produced, his decision on this question is clear: he unhesitatingly proclaimed his identity as a cripple and vowed to help crip pled children gain access to education. In publicizing himself as a 'cripple', Sullivan hoped to reshape the way in which both the disabled and the non-disabled defined the cripple. In other words, Sullivan sought to alter the existing disability discourse as it related to crippledom. His efforts included a consistent willingness to allow himself to be photographed while seated in his wheelchair, riding his hand-cranked bike, or in his goat-powered cart. In print, he unflinchingly described his physical condition in autobiographical articles, right down to the deformity in his hands caused by years of dragging himself about the floor of his family's home. Further, he never hesitated to draw upon anecdotes from his own life in order to call attention to the diffi-culties facing cripples. His candour concerning his physical flaws was hardly consistent with the cultural norms of the day. Some cripples, for instance, declined to sign their names to published articles detailing their experiences. Meanwhile, in certain municipalities the public display of physical impair-ments was a punishable offence (Burgdorf and Burgdorf 1980). Ryan (1990) cites a very early example of so-called 'ugly laws' preventing crippled beggars from displaying disfigured limbs. The motivation behind such laws, according to Ryan, seems to have been to avoid upsetting the supposedly delicate sensibilities of women. Given the climate of the times, Sullivan's frankness was not only remarkable, but demonstrated a certain pride in his self-identity and a desire to alter the public discourse concerning the cripple.

Sullivan also challenged the existing discourse in more direct ways. In fact, Sullivan appropriated the term 'cripple' for his own purposes, redefining it to suit his goals and aspirations for those with whom he shared, in his own words, 'a tie that binds' (1918b: 8–9). In the later nineteenth and early twen tieth century, most Americans seem to have viewed the so-called cripple as an object of pity, and thus the rightful heir to charity. The public image of the cripple was tied to charity through literary works such as Dickens's *Christmas Carol*, as well as through public policy such as Civil War pensions for disabled veterans and laws establishing the cripple's right to beg. Sullivan rejected the nineteenth-century linkage connecting the cripple to pity and unorganized charity, arguing that these twin evils were primarily responsible for the appalling conditions facing crippled children. On a daily basis, Sullivan argued (1923a: 3), the young cripple faced a 'stifling pity . . . murderous to his very nature'. Equally ruinous was what Sullivan referred to as the 'old way' of dispensing charity, in which dupes simply gave 'bread and meat' to those in need. 'The old way is destructive,' he proclaimed, 'and its wide practice is what has given a black eye to organized charity.' The 'new way', on the other hand, involved 'furnishing a ladder by which' the needy could 'climb up and out of the valley of vagrancy and need' (1921b: 6). Initially, education served as the ladder which Sullivan proposed – the tool by which the cripple could climb above the social and cultural barriers of American society. To this end, he edited at least three different journals, published hundreds of his own articles, and travelled the country advocating the creation of educational and medical institutions for crippled children.

Sullivan's efforts would likely have triggered little response during the nineteenth century. Yet the progressive era brought with it a reform discourse focusing on the theme of efficiency which meshed well with Sullivan's own arguments. This discourse emphasized a programme based on the limited and prudent spending of charitable dollars. Direct aid of any sort was generally abhorred. Between roughly 1890 and 1920, reformers obsessed with making society more efficient decried the unorganized system of charity characteristic of the nineteenth century. In words that echoed Sullivan's words, they decried the effects of charity upon the individual, claiming that a criminal and mendicant class had emerged from 'foolish philanthropists aided by an over-generous and soft-hearted public'. Progressive reformers proposed a 'systematic' approach to charity administered by knowledgeable authorities capable of discriminating between the 'worst kinds' of beggars and the 'industrious and deserving poor' (Bentwick 1894: 128). As Alice Willard Solenberger (1911) pointed out in her influential study entitled *One Thousand Homeless Men*, cripples and other disabled people were central to the problem of unorganized charity. Years of dependency created men whom she referred to as 'parasitic cripples', individuals in whom years of unemployment had seeded a permanent aversion to work. Worse still, these individuals served as a constant drain on the American economy. The solution to eliminating the inefficiency in the American economy created by indiscriminate charity involved not only a more careful management of expenditures, but also finding jobs for the unemployed. Progressives demonstrated a remarkable confidence in the ability of the industrial economy to absorb all workers willing to put forth effort – including cripples (Rodgers 1978). Yet those espousing the rhetoric of efficiency added validity and force to Sullivan's arguments that cripples could be more than objects of pity and charity. By 1918, this idea had become so widely accepted that one reform-minded individual could claim, without censure, that the only cripple incapable of work 'is a deliberate shirker' (Kaufman 1918: 22).

In some ways, the strategies Sullivan developed mirrored the methods of more recent disability rights activists, particularly in his rejection of pity (Gartner and Joe 1986; Shapiro 1993). Most importantly, Sullivan demonstrated a limited understanding of how disability was both socially and culturally constructed. He clearly understood that physical barriers such as stairs, or cultural barriers such as the devaluation of a disabled individual's abilities, created greater obstacles to employment and other social functions than actual physical impairment. Rather than seeing crippled children as devoid of potential, Sullivan's life experiences convinced him that all cripples maintained the potential for success similar to his own. In fact, he argued that children with disabilities could not only compete with non-disabled children academically, but held a 'mental superiority' over the non-disabled child – a superiority resulting from what he referred to as 'The Law of Compensation' (1919: 8), borrowing from the concept developed by Emerson (Sullivan 1919: 3). 'The great sufferings of crippledom' had little to do with one's 'physical condition', but rather emanated from 'a social arrangement that virtually condemns the cripple to mendicancy' (1919: 4). Without the realization that disability is most importantly a product of the physical and cultural barriers created by non-disabled society, it would have been difficult, if not impossible, for Sullivan to argue for the child's right to an education. Since individual misfortune provides weak ground for the establishment of civil rights, it was crucial that Sullivan put forth a definition of cripples as something more than physically impaired individuals.

Repeatedly, Sullivan argued that 'it is the crippled child's right to have an opportunity to enjoy the benefits that accrue from our public school system'. The crippled child was deserving of such rights, he concluded, 'not as an individual but as a class' (1919: 8). As a class, crippled children deserved either the modification of existing schools or the creation of new schools to create an unrestricted environment with such features as 'accessible lavatories, low blackboards, elevators for wheelchairs and crutches, adjustable seats' and even 'a specially designed and equipped gymnasium'. Sullivan's earliest efforts at raising awareness of the discrimination facing crippled children demonstrates a somewhat radical critique of American society. In his book *The Unheard Cry*, Sullivan used such words as 'murder' to describe the treatment of cripples in American society, and held that Americans did not recognize cripples as 'real, vibrating humans' (1914: 63).

Soon after the publication of *The Unheard Cry*, Sullivan joined a growing reform movement seeking to aid the crippled child. On his own, Sullivan agitated almost exclusively for access to education. As part of a larger progressive reform movement, however, he joined in calling for the establishment of institutions capable of delivering a combination of medicine and education. These institutions were most appropriately referred to by contemporaries as 'hospital-schools'. Over the 30-year span from 1900 to 1930, reformers, medical doctors and educators constructed some 70 institutions in the United States fitting the hospital school mode. Hospital-schools ranged in size from modest facilities of less than 30 'pupil-patients', to large institutions with hundreds of beds. Though diverse in their physical structure and even in name (only about one-third were actually referred to as hospital-schools), they shared a common commitment to preparing the crippled child for entrance into the mainstream of America's workaday world through the application of both medical treatment and education (Solenberger 1914; Abt 1924). After he accepted a position as the educational director (and unofficial spokesperson) for the Van Leuven Browne Hospital School in Detroit, Sullivan's rhetoric took a new course. Once committed exclusively to the education of crippled children, Sullivan now became a spokesman for an institution that would soon become chiefly a medical centre.

Sullivan never relented in his calls for legislators to establish the cripple's right to an education, but nevertheless made crucial mistakes within his discourse which limited the success of his life's work. The more minor of the two flaws involved an apparent confusion on the part of Sullivan between 'duty' and 'rights'. His strongest argument for the rights of the cripple to an education appear in an article reprinted in several educational journals simply titled 'The crippled child's rights' (Sullivan 1919). In this article, Sullivan argues that the cripple has a guaranteed right to an education. By arguing in terms of rights, Sullivan resolved that the cripple deserved the same opportunities as any member of society. Yet in numerous other articles, including one written only months prior to his forceful call for the rights of the crippled child, Sullivan argued in a somewhat different vein. On these occasions, he claimed it was the 'duty' of the state to provide care for 'the afflicted' (1918a: 4). This latter argument harked back to the nineteenth-century discourse Sullivan and other progressives strove to replace. In his article, Sullivan drew upon a speech by Abraham Lincoln in which Lincoln proclaimed it the state's duty to provide, 'in every way possible', for 'the delinquent, defective and dependent' classes. Here, Sullivan made not only the unfortunate mistake of linking cripples to the poor and criminal – a common nineteenth-century connection that many progressives, including Sullivan, sought to sever – but also, by speaking in terms of duty and obligation, subverted his claims to guaranteed rights. In such ways, Sullivan sent forth conflicting messages: that on the one hand crippled children were capable of competing with non-disabled children on a level playing field, but on the other hand they deserved the paternalistic protection of the state. It also demonstrated that Sullivan himself was willing to accept something less than guaranteed rights.

A more significant mistake was Sullivan's joining forces with a medical establishment committed to the defining of cripples as individuals whose primary problem was physical impairment. Sullivan, along with other reformers working to offer crippled children a better future, readily allied their efforts with those of orthopaedic surgery. This move once again reflected the tendency of disability discourse to become entangled with the larger discourses of the day. Where the progressive discourse involving efficiency meshed relatively well with Sullivan's arguments, another, the progressive faith in all things scientific, created an obstacle to the establishment of disability civil rights that remains in place today. This faith led progressives to an easy acceptance of claims by both medical and non-medical 'experts' that orthopaedic surgery could eliminate crippledom. Sullivan's tacit acceptance of the orthopedist's authority subverted his own assertion that cripples were a group deserving of civil rights. As the orthopaedic profession gained in prestige and became an accepted, if somewhat marginal, medical speciality, efforts to alleviate crippled children became increasingly tied to the orthopaedist's mission to cure. This grandiose, if futile, plan left little room for Sullivan's educational mission.

Further, as the sociologist Robert Bogdan argues, the medicalization of disability resulted in 'the growth of organized charities, the rise of professional fund-raising, and the invention of the poster child, with *pity* used as the dominant mode of presenting human difference' (Bogdan 1988: 278). During the 1920s and 1930s, massive amounts of money poured into curative efforts, while the progressive focus on educating crippled children lost momentum. Wealthy philanthropists such as Detroit's James Couzens donated millions to the construction of children's orthopaedic hospitals, while making little or no provision for the continued education of the children. In the early 1920s, the fraternal organization known commonly as the Shriners began establishing dozens of orthopaedic hospitals across the nation, while in the 1930s the Roosevelt-inspired March of Dimes began annual fund-raising which would produce millions of dollars for polio research and medical treatment. These and other charitable efforts painted a very different picture of the crippled child than did progressives. The understanding of crippled children as individuals to be not consoled but encouraged deteriorated in the face of pity-driven fund-raising campaigns. In fact, Sullivan was not oblivious of the problems of linking a campaign for the education of crippled children to one driven by a search for a cure. In 1923, Sullivan posed the question in the *Detroit News*, 'Should the state see to the hospitalization of the crippled child in preference to his education?' The question arose as Sullivan realized that the demand for state money to fund hospitals had subsequently resulted in a dearth of funding for educational efforts. A large reason for Michigan's failure to establish schools, Sullivan realized, was the common misconception that orthopaedists could quickly cure all cripples of their physical impairments – a belief which Sullivan helped instil in the legislature through his promotion of the Michigan Hospital-School. Now Sullivan was forced to admit that 'The process of treating, much less curing crippled children is a slow one – many times requiring years of constant care and observation of surgeons', and that 'another large per cent' will never be cured (1923b: 11). Yet while Sullivan was willing to admit limitations to the healing abilities of orthopaedists, he could not bring himself to criticize a profession in which he not only placed tremendous confidence, but on whose (albeit limited) 'healing abilities' his livelihood depended. Ultimately, however, Sullivan's argument that crippled children had the right to accessible schools began to sound hollow in the context of a journal increasingly filled with medical reports and calls for public donations to aid cripples.

The progressive emphasis on efficiency and science each impacted the evolving disability discourse in profound ways. Initially, the 'gospel of efficiency', as one historian has referred to the progressive obsession with efficiency, led to a discourse rejecting the association of the cripple with pity and charity. Yet it was the progressive affinity for science, and particularly for medical science, which had the more permanent impact upon disability discourse. What Sullivan and other educational reformers apparently failed to understand was that by linking their reform goals to medicine they spread the seeds for the failure of their own hopes and dreams.

# 17

# Art and lies? Representations of disability on film

## Tom Shakespeare

### Introduction

From its early days, the disabled people's movement has focused attention on the power of images to define the experience of impairment, and to foster prejudicial attitudes towards disabled people. A range of British and American writers have indicated the dominance of stereotypes of tragedy, evil and incapacity in various media, perhaps especially focusing on film (Longmore 1987; Morris 1991; Sutherland 1996; Darke 1998b). As a recent survey of the past century of cinema indicated, crudely distorted discourses of disability have been ubiquitous since the very earliest days (Norden 1994).

To summarize a large and growing literature, the main problems with mainstream representations of disabled people are that such characters are usually objectified and distanced from the audience. Their particular impairment is made the most important thing about the person. The character usually slips into one of three major stereotypes: the tragic but brave invalid (for example, Tiny Tim); the sinister cripple (for example, Dr No); the 'supercrip', who has triumphed over tragedy (for example, Helen Keller). The dominant plot devices often centre either on the desire of the physically impaired character for revenge against the world (*Freaks, Acción Mutante*), or the attempt at cure of the impairment, often assisted by a non-disabled teacher, doctor or therapist. The role of such characters and plots is to provide highly visual *hooks*, to engage the audience's interest, whether via sympathy or revulsion. The disabled character is therefore a means to an end, a vehicle through which the film-maker can enable viewers to discharge emotion and become involved in the story. It is very rare for a disabled character to be featured who does not have such a role: incidental disabled characters in other roles are very infrequent, and in instances where disabled people are seen as extras or background characters, this is intended to heighten an atmosphere of exoticism, perversion, evil or fantasy.

Disabled viewers and critics have condemned this historical distortion of disability, and quite rightly so. The use of disability as character trait, plot device, or as atmosphere is a lazy short-cut. These representations are not accurate or fair reflections of the actual experience of disabled people. Such stereotypes reinforce negative attitudes towards disabled people, and ignorance about the nature of disability. Very often, the roles themselves are played by non-disabled people, and the critical reception of such performances centres on the ability of the actor to mimic the supposed behavioural characteristics of people with such impairments. Above all, the dominant images are crude, one-dimensional and simplistic.

My argument in this chapter, however, is that the legitimate critique of what Norden has called 'the cinema of isolation', and what Darke has labelled 'normality drama', is in danger of being extended into simplistic and overcensorious readings of almost every film including impairment. In a parallel to some excesses associated with Political Correctness, a new Disability Correctness is undermining the possibility of film-makers dealing with impairment at all. While it is appropriate to critique simplistic and one-dimensional representations of disability, it is too easy to reject complex and nuanced works of film art which do not comply with politically charged notions of 'positive imagery'. There is a dangerous willingness to take offence at supposed violations of equality principles. Moreover, the desire for a positive representation can obscure the elements of cliché and distortion in films which are heralded as 'good' portrayals. A more sophisticated approach to reading films is needed, which engages with the film-maker's intentions, and achieves a balanced appraisal of the outcome.

I will try and demonstrate this argument through a discussion of two prominent recent cinematic treatments of disability. First, I will offer a neutral summary of plot, drawn from the film periodical *Sight and Sound*. Then I will summarize the response of disabled reviewers. Subsequently I will offer my own reading of the films, before concluding with general comments about representations of disability.

## The films

*Breaking the Waves* and *Shine* were two highly acclaimed award-winning films of 1996, distinguished by their melodramatic stories and superb acting. Both were controversial due to their disability themes, and they were received very differently by the disability community.

*Breaking the Waves*, written and directed by Danish director Lars Von Trier (1996), won the Grand Prix at Cannes and was widely praised in film journals. Set in the 1970s, it concerns the 'naive' Bess, who lives in a strict Presbyterian community in north-west Scotland, and marries Jan, a Norwegian oil-rig worker. Despite the disapproval of the elders, all goes well until Jan returns to the rigs and Bess is 'driven to distraction'. Her prayers to God for Jan's return are 'answered cruelly' when Jan returns after an accident, seemingly paralysed from the neck down. Her best friend is worried about Bess's mental stability, but the village doctor does not believe she is mentally ill.

Jan suggests to Bess that she takes a lover, and later tries to commit suicide. Back in hospital, he insists that Bess takes a lover, in order to tell him about it. She resists and he continues to deteriorate. After she masturbates a stranger on a bus, Jan seems to improve. She then works as a prostitute, and is ostracized from the community: the village doctor advises Jan to have her sectioned, but Bess escapes from hospital. On hearing that Jan is dying, she visits the ship of a sadistic sailor and is beaten and cut. Back at the hospital, she discovers Jan is no better, and she dies. At the coroner's enquiry she is pathologized, and the elders refuse her a funeral service. Jan, now largely recovered, steals her body with the aid of his friends, and they give her a burial at sea. Later that night, he is woken by his companions: in mid-ocean, in bright moonlight, the sky is full of the sound of pealing bells.

*Shine* was described by *Sight and Sound* as 'real life melodrama', and Geoffrey Rush won the Best Actor Oscar for his portrayal of David Helfgott, a brilliant piano student who 'suffered' a mental breakdown. Director Scott Hicks subtly associates David's mental illness with his father's experience of the Holocaust. The film opens in Australia in the 1980s, as the eccentric and middle-aged David taps on the door of a restaurant, and is befriended by Sylvia. Flashing back to the 1950s, we see the young piano prodigy being pushed by Peter, his father. He becomes successful, but is consistently put under pressure by his disturbed father, although he is encouraged and supported by others. Forbidden by Peter to go to the United States, he finally breaks with his father and goes to London to study. Performing Rachmaninov's Third Piano Concerto, he collapses.

Back in Australia, he lives in a care-home, until one of the helpers befriends him and takes him in as a lodger. There he starts playing the piano again. After meeting Sylvia in the restaurant, he begins playing for the diners. He moves in with Sylvia and meets her friend Gillian, an astrologer. When David proposes, Gillian realizes that their partnership is astrologically intended. They marry, and her support enables him to become a performer again. In his dreams, he is reconciled with his father.

**The critical response**

The two films under discussion received a markedly dichotomous response from the British disability media. Reviewing *Shine*, Andy Kimpton-Nye (1997: 18) used phrases such as 'expertly crafted bio-pic', 'moving', and 'I loved it'. He suggested that 'deft and subtle plotting', positioned impairment as 'integral' to the storyline, 'not as sensational subject matter simply dished up for its "exoticness" or freak show factor'. Moreover there were all-round 'awesome performances'. The conclusion, showing Helfgott established in the community through access to employment and support from friends and loved ones, was regarded by this reviewer as very positive.

The following month, reviewer Lois Keith went so far as to contrast *Shine*, 'the best film I've seen for ages', with *Breaking the Waves*, which she felt was 'one of the worst' (Keith 1997: 16): she stated that 'I found almost everything I saw on the screen unbelievably mysogynist [*sic*], oppressive and above all, cliched.' For Keith, the representation of disability, and the representation of women, were irredeemably prejudiced. In her reading, Jan had become paralysed by his accident, 'the classic picture of the bitter, self-hating cripple'; Bess was mentally fragile, becoming mentally ill, and the whole story was to be read as a stereotypical drama of cure. Echoing Paul Darke, she concluded that 'we must never underestimate the power of the cliché. Nor how attractive to the public imagination is the idea that you can be paralysed by a wish or a misdeed, redeemed by the power of love and cured.'

In a subsequent month, *DAIL* published a letter from mental-health survivor Peter Rose, who challenged this author's more positive reading of the film, and criticized what he saw as the traditional stereotype of the mentally ill person as being 'simple but closer to God' (Rose 1997: 12). In *Disability Now*, Michael Turner had also described Bess as schizophrenic, suggesting that the film's plot was 'as exploitative of disabled people as any low brow slasher movie' (Turner 1996: 19). While Turner did highlight the importance of the religious setting, and the affirmation of love against a background of repression, he also used words like 'perverse' and 'unlikely' to describe Jan's request for Bess to seek alternative sexual experiences, and concluded that the message was that 'love is only possible with sex and that disabled people are unable to attain either'.

At the end of the year, these dominant political readings of the films were reinforced in the annual 'Raspberry Ripple' awards, for positive and negative representations of disability. *Shine* was positively cited for its images of mental illness, and won the Best Film category, while *Breaking the Waves* was nominated under the category of Worst Film.

## Alternative readings

I wish to argue that shallow readings and Disability Correctness have led to misleading evaluations of both films. First, I concur with Maria Oshodi, whose letter to *DAIL* went against the tide of positive receptions of the Helfgott biopic: 'What is all this eulogising over Shine? The film I witnessed bowed low at the altar of cliché, especially the snoringly typical scenario of Able-bodied Woman rising out of the mists at the end to save Disabled Man' (Oshodi 1997).

In her view, the film was fatuous, it negated the 'complexity of relationships' and it reinforced the stereotype of woman as carer. There are many similar films where a madman is saved by the love of a good woman, which usually have been lambasted by disabled critics.

Another critical comment came from Judy Singer, the mother of a child with Asperger's syndrome:

*Shine's* popularity is the last gasp (hopefully) of the psychotherapeutic notion that if there is any anomaly in the child's life, the parents are to blame. It's an exercise in parent bashing, and its popularity lies in the fervent hope of large sections of the population that every painful situation has a simple cause. From the point of view of myself and some other parents of children with marginal impairments, who are constantly under suspicion (just what did you do to make that child so whatever . . .,), far from being inspiring the film was depressing and infuriating.

(posting to the Internet)

She added that the sister of David Helfgott had come out angrily claiming that the depiction of their father was inaccurate.

*Shine* certainly played into the traditional view of 'tormented genius', particularly the passionate and unbalanced musician. Helfgott can be seen as the latest of a line of musical eccentrics, including Alfred Molina's BBC portrayal of John Ogden, and the film *Thirty Two Short Films about Glenn Gould*. The idea of an artist struggling with schizophrenia is familiar from films such as *An Angel at My Table*. In real life, it appears from the very mixed reception of his concert tour that David Helfgott is hardly the brilliant maestro that the film suggests. Indeed, making his character into a brilliant musician could be said to play into the conventional trope of 'compensatory abilities', just as Dustin Hoffman's autistic character in *Rain Man* had extraordinary arithmetical skills.

As with the *Rain Man* character, Helfgott is infantilized by his portrayal, in scenes such as the one where he bounces, semi-naked, on the trampoline. In this and other scenes, his enthusiasm, frenetic conversation, and lack of social skills cause other characters, and the audience, to laugh at him. He becomes an endearing, childish figure of fun, in the tradition of the cinematic 'Sweet Innocent' disabled figure identified by Norden. We are encouraged to admire his women friends' patience and tolerance of his eccentricities, and their roles are as mother-figures to Helfgott.

While the disability movement has praised the depiction of mental illness, the film operates entirely within a medical discourse of madness. While it could be seen to be positive, in the sense that the character is accepted, with his eccentricities, and there is a happy ending, this outcome is achieved by glossing over the political issues surrounding his illness. For example, we do not gain much insight into his incarceration in a nursing home, or his interactions with the medical profession. There is one scene where we discover he has been forbidden to play the piano, but no other clue as to his experience as a 'mental-health system survivor'. The notion that he is truly 'mad' is never challenged; rather it is suggested that it is okay to be 'mad' if you are (a) a musical genius and (b) looked after by a saintly female.

The acclaimed performances, again, could be said to follow the tradition whereby non-disabled actors are praised for their success in mimicking the tics and traits of people with mental or physical impairments. When Daniel Day-Lewis managed a tour-de-force impression of cerebral palsy in *My Left*

*Foot*, the film-makers were criticized for their use of a non-disabled actor; Hoffman and many other actors have similarly been viewed with scepticism by the disabled community when they apply method-acting to impairment roles. Yet, in the case of *Shine*, there seems to have been a collective suspension of critical disbelief.

It is not my intention entirely to demolish *Shine*, which undoubtedly had many strengths, particularly the overlooked performance of Noah Taylor as the young David. I merely wish to demonstrate that there are valid alternative readings. The sophistication with which the Holocaust issue was dealt with was not matched by its oversentimental treatment of disability, particularly the romantic element, and the plot line falls into many of the routine representational pitfalls. Somehow, disabled audiences have apparently accepted a film which is no marked improvement on the simplistic and shallow clichés of previous imagery.

In contrast to the one-dimensionality of *Shine*, I wish to argue that *Breaking the Waves* is a complex, ambitious and successful film, which does not have very much to do with disability at all, despite particular details. While *Shine* purports to be a realistic biographical portrayal, *Breaking the Waves* is clearly a work of fiction. Nor, contrary to disabled readings, is it centrally about sex, cure via the love of a good woman, or mental illness. Instead, it is a highly metaphorical, complex and resonant film about religion and redemption: the correlation is not so much *Lady Chatterley's Lover* as *Babette's Feast*.

The non-literal context of the film is signalled by the interset 'chapter headings', highly tinted island scenes, which seem to be stills until slight movement is detected. These are accompanied by ironic use of 1960s and 1970s pop classics – for instance, Procul Harum's *Whiter Shade of Pale* – on the soundtrack. Lars Von Trier described such interludes as a 'God's eye-view of the landscape in which the story is unfolding, as if he is watching over the characters'. While the use of *cinema verité*-style camera work implies realism, we are actually in the realm of symbol and parable, centring on love and sacrifice: the original title of the film was to be *Amor Omnie*, 'love is omnipresent'.

Bess's direct conversation with God is contrasted with the repressive, hypocritical and unforgiving Calvinism of the village elders. This is a film, as Von Trier has argued, where 'Religion is accused, but not God.' In the elders' Presbyterian world, women are marginalized and insignificant. They do not accept the existence of miracles, and do not even allow church bells. This Puritan rigidity is contrasted with the alternative, passionate, sensual approach to life: whereas in *Babette's Feast* the difference was food, here the difference is sex.

Bess's love of life and enjoyment of her sexuality is celebrated. Above all, the depth and unselfish nobility of her love for Jan ensure that ultimately she is redeemed. When she prays for her husband's return – echoes of W.W. Jacobs's *The Monkey's Paw* – she literally gets what she wants, although Jan is represented as being sick, rather than disabled (*pace* disabled reviewers). Nowhere is it suggested that he has broken his spine: rather the oil-rig accident seems to have caused a mysterious head injury. Neither is it firmly suggested that Bess is mentally ill. While her direct religiosity may appear insane to modern audiences, it is treated with dignity and respect by the film-maker. It is the disabled reviewers who have made the assumption of madness, reinforcing the medical discourse of insanity which is firmly challenged by the film.

Bess, in my reading, is certainly angelic, and implicitly a Christ-like figure. She is a thoroughly good person. Rejected by the religious authorities (paralleling the Scribes and Pharisees of the Gospels), she experiences humiliation and physical torture. She gives her body in order that others might live, sacrificing her life for that of others. Although she dies as a result, at a later stage we see that she is redeemed – that her love has been recognized – when the Heavens open and the bells ring, symbolizing her union with God, and his approval of her behaviour.

The problem with the critical reception of *Breaking the Waves* by disabled reviewers has been the way that this non-realist film has been judged by realist criteria. For example, it would be like criticizing the portrayal of alcoholic hallucination in *Harvey*. Yet in *Harvey*, the audience is eventually brought to understand that James Stewart is 'actually' seeing a six-foot rabbit: in the world of the film, the Pooka exists. Similarly, in *Breaking the Waves*, miracles do happen and God does speak directly to the world. Comments such as 'unlikely' show that reviewers are reading the film literally, rather than engaging with its metaphor and symbolism.

The film is clearly more complex and more problematic than the reading I have offered: Jan's misconceived suggestion that Bess continues her erotic development via sex with others, which appears to be intended to be read as an unselfish sacrifice, is misguided (perhaps under the influence of his medication). So is the literal way in which Bess carries out his suggestion. However, they both act through love: both their intentions are good. We are not meant to feel comfortable with Bess's faith, or her sacrifice, despite the miraculous redemption. As Lizzie Francke (1996) argued in *Sight and Sound*, *Breaking the Waves* 'strives to understand goodness' but it is as if 'our very faith in the film is meant to be shaken'. It is a disturbing, almost horrific film, but I think this is an intentional part of its role as an authentic work of art.


## Conclusion

By exploring these two films, I have demonstrated that disability discourses are more complex and multi-faceted than might appear. While there can be a basic consensus about ways in which images can be exploitative and stereotyping, it is dangerous to develop hard and fast rules of representation, against which the disability credentials of a particular film can be read off straightforwardly. While disabled activists, like feminists and others, always have the right to condemn specific treatments, it is unduly prescriptive and censorious to draw up narrow criteria of what constitutes 'correct' imagery, and this only serves to limit artistic creativity. Approaching a film prepared to take offence or be insulted is not a good starting point for critique.

I am not proposing that whereas mainstream films – a James Bond block-buster or a Disney film like *The Hunchback of Notre Dame* – should be criticized for resorting to stereotype, avant-garde or art house films should be exempt from criticism. There is a long list of 'arty', usually pretentious, films which reproduce crude and unthinking distortions of disability (for example, *Boxing Helena*). Short-cuts to empathy or alienation are employed by both the alternative auteurs and conventional Hollywood directors. It would be unwise for disabled critics to go down the parallel path to those who have labelled mass-market sex images 'pornographic' and up-market sex images 'erotic'.

A film, like any text, can be read in different ways. However, authorial intentions have a crucial role in conditioning our response to a work of art, and we should engage with what the artist is trying to do, and then judge the extent to which s/he has succeeded. Jumping to conclusions, on the basis of superficial elements of plot and characterization, is not to do justice to any work of narrative art. Equally, film is an art form, not a literal representation of reality, and demands to be judged on artistic elements, not simply verisimilitude. All critical responses will be subjective, but we should be able to decide personally that we dislike a film, while making a more objective appraisal of its strengths and weaknesses.

A critical position which is unduly reductive, simplistic, or based on one criterion alone does not seem to be a worthy enterprise. For example, from a Marxist perspective, bourgeois novels like those of Jane Austen or Marcel Proust seem entirely redundant and based on economic exploitation and class privilege. Yet as works of art, they are undeniably well-written and insightful, and there is a broad consensus about their lasting value. Similarly, it would be possible to reject *The Merchant of Venice* for its anti-Semitism, or *King Lear* for its portrait of madness, or *Richard III* for its equation of moral and physical impairment. Yet these plays have also great complexity, depth and value. It is possible to fail on one criterion, yet succeed on others.

We should approach a work of art with a range of questions: is it well made and well performed? Are the characters complex or shallow? Is the plot engaging or predictable? Is the message nuanced or trite? We are likely to conclude with a mixed appraisal, which finds fault with particular elements, and is more or less impressed by other areas. The traditional, prejudiced, representations of disability usually occur in contexts in which the judgement on most of these criteria is very negative: films are not good at portraying disability in particular, because they are not good films in general. In some other examples, a good film is marred by the crudity of the disabled content. We need to attempt a balanced evaluation of the overall work, which does not ignore disability issues, but does not judge solely on the basis of this element, except perhaps in the crudest cases. As a parallel, we might say that D.W. Griffith's *Birth of a Nation* is almost entirely undermined by its racist elements, despite its historical and technical value, whereas *Gone with the Wind* succeeds despite its dubious racial features and context.

A film like *Breaking the Waves* requires more work on the part of an audience than a film like *Shine*. There is more going on in the film, more originality, more ambiguity: shades of grey rather than black and white. The more complex, subtle and nuanced a work of art is, the better chance it has to achieve greatness. On this criterion, I would argue that *Breaking the Waves* is a deep film, undoubtedly of great artistic merit, which has been unfairly judged by the disability community, who have been unwilling to engage with the message about religion and redemption. In contrast, *Shine* is a good but slight film, whose merits in terms of disability discourse have been over-stated. It aspires to romanticism, but achieves only sentimentality.

In the context of a brief review in *Disability Now* or *DAIL* it is difficult to develop sophisticated judgements. But the shallowness of the critiques under discussion parallels a lack of aesthetic engagement in the disability community as a whole. Personal distaste for a particular film is made the basis for a sweeping political and artistic dismissal. Yet there is a need for broader debate about disabling representations. While the common problems of stereotypes have been identified, there is less consensus about what consti-tutes a 'positive image'. If disabled activists want the broad message about prejudice to be taken on board by the film industry, and artists in general, then it may be necessary to take a more positive and less one-dimensional view of representation, lest we are accused of failing to see the wood for the trees, or even of being prejudiced ourselves.

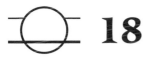 **18**

# What they don't tell disabled people with learning difficulties

**Simone Aspis**

## Introduction

The 1990 NHS and Community Care Act placed emphasis on disabled people having greater choices and increased participation and involvement in the planning of community care. It became increasingly important for service agencies to provide information about their services to disabled people, in particular those who had been labelled as having learning difficulties. Since this Act was passed, jargon-free information provision has also become a feature of health and educational institutions. As a result, 'accessible' information packs on a wide range of subjects related to independent living, community care, rights and speaking up for disabled people with the learning difficulties label have flooded the information market. This has seemingly represented a wider recognition of the importance of providing information using jargon-free language; but in the disability field, such materials are promoted, and often praised, as enabling effective communication with, and therefore empowerment of, disabled people with the learning difficulties label. Close examination of these materials should therefore allow us to determine how effective this jargon-free information is in its goal of empowerment, what exactly is being communicated and who it is being communicated to. This is important because a major part of empowerment is how language is used in creating and advocating social change. This chapter makes a critical examination of recent jargon-free materials targeted at disabled people with the learning difficulties label. It argues that a number of outstanding issues need to be addressed if the information is to achieve its stated goals.

**Language**

It is first important to explain what I mean by two terms which are used throughout this chapter – *disabled people with the learning difficulties label* and *jargon*.

I usually describe myself as a disabled person who has been labelled by the system as having learning difficulties. This makes it very clear that the name, and the identity 'learning difficulty', have been *imposed* on me by the system, in particular, the education system which pre-defines 'learning ability'. There is a great deal of research which supports this view. For example:

> One invented modern category – which definitely invokes 'normality' – is 'mental retardation' (in the US) or 'learning difficulties' (in the UK). While once some individuals were seen as 'half-witted', 'dunces', 'a bit slow', or whatever, a distinct population category has been created out of the diffuse individual diversity of intellectual (in)competences. This category's coherence derives primarily from the exclusionary treatment of its members, and the services delivered to them on the basis of their categorisation (Trent 1995). Research in the USA by Mehan *et al.* (1986) and Mercer (1973) suggests that testing may be pre-eminently influential in the construction of individual educational careers and identities as 'mentally retarded'.
>
> (Jenkins 1996: 167, and references therein)

'Learning difficulties' are also created by examination systems which label, categorize and segregate children who do not acquire prescribed knowledge, learn and solve problems in a set way within a time limit set by non-disabled people. Testing and examination systems use the label 'learning difficulty' as a self-fulfilling philosophy. Once a child is labelled in this way it becomes almost impossible to change the image the label creates because teaching and learning are geared to reinforcing it by making everything simple – and therefore leaving a lot of information out – so that disabled people with the learning difficulties label 'can understand it'. The label therefore not only assumes that a person is only capable of limited thinking and knowledge acquisition but requires that this assumption is *reflected* in the educational materials they are exposed to.

These systems and assumptions which both exclude and disable me are part of my oppression as a *disabled person*, this term indicating that I am also a part of a movement which is made up of people who seek social change collectively. If these systems were abolished then comparisons between disabled and non-disabled children on the basis of intellectual ability would disappear, which would in turn remove the negative consequences of labelling, categorizing and segregation. I feel this is true for all children with what professionals describe as having 'specific and general learning difficulties'.

*Jargon* refers to two areas of language. Firstly, it refers to language which is not in the vocabulary of a particular group of people and is left unexplained.

This is important because all language is open to interpretation and the English language is based on shades of subtlety and vagueness. If jargon is misused, there is an increased risk that the content of the message will be misunderstood or ignored. I think that language which is implicitly or explicitly used by or which influences the lives of the *general population*, such as the language of the law, policies and contracts, should be made available in jargon-free language. Without this, jargon simply reinforces the power and authority of the professionals who use it: politicians, local authority officials, lawyers and educational psychologists, for example. Complicated and ambiguous legal language simply ensures that ordinary people do not fully understand their legal rights, and this may deny them the quality of life to which the law says they are entitled. In such circumstances, free access to documents of legislation in local libraries, for example, is just a token gesture which ultimately works *against* the protection of people's rights.

A distinction needs to be made between this kind of jargon and the subtleties and specialities within the English language, though there are ways in which both can lead to maintaining the status quo and reinforcing existing power relationships. There is a place for specialist language which explains new ideas which cannot be explained using existing language; in some walks of life, such as the academic world, the ability to use this language effectively symbolizes status and often determines how successful someone can be. But language that begins in a specialist field often moves into the general population. For example, Mike Oliver notes, in relation to disability, that

> the application of [the social model of disability] to particular issues and contexts seemed outdated both in terms of the language used and because the world had moved on; new legislation, new organisations, new methods of action and so on.

> (Oliver 1996a: 1–2)

Another example might be the language of computing. Specialist words such as 'megabyte', 'RAM', 'DOS' and 'floppy disc' were developed at a time when only a few people had access to computers. But as computers become part of many households in the Western world, and children increasingly use them in schools, there is a need to explain these words in simpler, more accessible language. When this specialist language moves into more general use, so that it becomes part of everyday vocabulary – as the social model now is both within and outside the disability movement – it may nevertheless be used as a short cut, that is, to *avoid* explaining new concepts to those for whom the language is still inaccessible.

Disabled people themselves use both specialist language and jargon for various reasons which include explaining new ideas, trying to get on an equal footing with non-disabled stakeholders and holding power over other groups of people. Because the disability movement includes people with the learning difficulty label it becomes much more difficult to strike a balance between making sure that this language is accessible and overcoming the fear that non-disabled stakeholders will trivialize the concepts and ideas behind the language in a way which reinforces their own negative interpretations of disability and disabled people. This may be why Oliver goes on to say that:

> It may be true that I do not always communicate my ideas as clearly as I might, understanding disability requires a great deal of intellectual effort. If we are going to transform ourselves and society, it is only we as disabled people who can do the necessary intellectual work. Therefore ... while I try to communicate with clarity, I refuse to oversimplify the complexity of the ideas and issues which produce disability in the late twentieth century.
>
> (Oliver 1996a: 2–3)

I suspect this may be one reason why there has not been anything published on disability philosophies using jargon-free language.

## Power relationships

When understanding how groups of oppressed people are treated unfairly, it is essential to appreciate and to question the level of power that different groups of people have in their lives. Many people with learning difficulties have very little power because we have been taught to be dependent on state benefits, community care services and the personal and professional judgements and decisions of other people. The low levels of income we receive do limit our economic independence which, in turn, limits the amount of choice we have in our lives. Our autonomy is often directly influenced by the (in)flexibility of professional service providers. In 1996 the Open University worked with Mencap and People First to design a course which explores issues for disabled people with the learning difficulties label and their carers. This resulted in the production of a study pack *Learning Disability: Working as Equal People* (Open University 1996). The title of the study pack promotes the idea that equality between disabled people with the learning difficulties label and other groups of people already exists or, at least, is an ideal which can be aimed for – 'Equal partnership is when both people are equal, there is no boss, and there is trust and respect' (p. 10). This definition of equal partnership does not refer to the fact that partnership commonly consists of people having equal say and influence in implementing decisions made and in accessing resources. However, the imbalance of power, and therefore the types of decisions which disabled people with the learning difficulties label and other groups of people can make, has not been acknowledged. This is emphasized by some of the examples given to illustrate the concept of 'equal partnership': 'Pat Moffat, my social worker. We worked together for me to move home and job' (p. 28). 'May is the house parent in the hostel where I live. We work together so that our hostel is a comfortable place to live ...' (p. 28).

These examples do not say that the social worker carries out the community care assessment, writes up the care plan, and decides whether there are enough financial resources to provide the necessary support needed. If the social worker decides that the person needs a different form of accommodation or is not eligible for support then the client has to do without. With this knowledge, can these examples be described as 'equal partnership'? It is the social worker who has the power to influence the client's care assessment and whether the support will be provided by the local authority. The second example reduces 'equal partnership' to a practical level in order to suggest autonomy, but at the same time, seems not to refer to *who* makes decisions about what is 'comfortable'. Again, it is usually the house parents and other staff who make decisions about the accommodation policies and rules, how the household budget will be spent, employment of staff, and admission and eviction of residents. Residents often only influence decisions of a minor nature, such as the decor of the accommodation – which is possibly what is meant by making the hostel 'a comfortable place to live'. Even though there may appear to be partnership between the house parent and resident when helping to make the accommodation more comfortable, the fact remains that the house parent has the power to influence whether and how the relevant work is carried out. Thus, in both examples, it feels as if there is a 'boss', and disabled people with the learning difficulties label are taught to respect and trust professionals and staff because they are the 'boss'.

If *Learning Disability: Working as Equal People* had begun from a base which acknowledged *unequal* partnerships then this would have enabled a closer examination of how much power service providers and local authorities have over the lives of disabled people with the learning difficulties label, and how these decisions are influenced by political decisions made by central government which themselves are often based on dominant attitudes existing in society. Using the language of 'equal partnership' leaves the power relationships between disabled people with the learning difficulties label and other groups of people intact; dominant cultural attitudes are left unquestioned and unchallenged. Even when there is acknowledgement about the imbalance of power between disabled people with the learning difficulties label and other groups of people, there is still often an emphasis on sharing on equal terms:

> The word power in relation to people with learning difficulties can strike fear and trepidation into the hearts of staff, family, parents and even advisors. But if we are talking about genuine partnership with people with learning difficulties, then we must talk about power and face up to this challenge.
>
> (Whittaker 1991: 10)

There is no acknowledgement of when disabled people with the learning difficulties label *should* have more power than other groups of people. For example in self-advocacy groups, people with learning difficulties should have more power than the advisors. Consider a further example from the Open University pack (1996: 37) which concerns Gary, who is living on his own in the community supported by a team of support workers.

Gary gets:

- a home of his own;
- people to keep him company and take him out;
- help with day-to-day living;
- help to live how he wants to.

In this example it is not made clear whether Gary is the 'boss' and has the power to make decisions about the employment of staff, policies and rules in his home and whether, if the staff do not conform to his expectations, they lose the following privileges which come with the job.

The staff get:

- a paid job or a place to live;
- Gary's company – which they seem to enjoy;
- trips out with Gary to places they like – such as the pub and jazz evenings.

Within this concept of 'equal partnership' there is an implied assumption that disabled people with the learning difficulties label will always need to depend on non-disabled people who are in positions of power.

## History

This imbalance of power between disabled people and non-disabled people can be traced back into history. The current power that service providers, local authorities and governments have over our lives can be explained by the unchallenged power that similar people have had throughout history. There is correspondingly very little recognition of significant events which have occurred in the lives of disabled people with the learning difficulties label.

A recent People First publication, *Not Just Painted On*, aims to explain Down's syndrome and the rights which Down's syndrome people should have. It begins with this description:

> We are all made up of things called cells. These are like building bricks that make up our bodies. Cells are very small and can only be seen under a microscope. Cells are made up of even smaller things called Chromosomes. Most people have 46 chromosomes in each of their cells. People with Downs Syndrome have an extra chromosome in their cells. They have 47 chromosomes.
>
> (Perez *et al*. 1996: 5)

This description legitimates the medical profession's labelling and categorizing of people who are physically and intellectually different from what is 'expected' or what is seen to be 'normal' (people who have 46 chromosomes). This kind of medical definition was challenged in Chris Gooding's book about parents of Down's syndrome children. In the introduction Gooding explains:

Dr Down thought that the people at the bottom end of the scale of intelligence might have a different physical appearance from the rest [of society]. At the institution for the 'idiots' and 'insane' where he worked, he looked for individuals who might fit the bill and prove his theory right . . . The hospital was so large and so crammed with inmates that he was under pressure from the hospital management to classify them under different labels so that the bureaucracy could cope with organising them.

(Gooding 1991: x)

Using historical evidence, Gooding suggests that the Down's syndrome label originated in mechanisms of social control. What is striking is that nowhere in any of the jargon-free publications produced by People First is this possibility acknowledged in the definitions given of learning difficulties or disability. Indeed, there is a consistent failure to define 'disability' and 'learning difficulty', an omission which implies acceptance of existing definitions and allows powerful groups of people to continue to define our experience using the 'accepted' and now commonplace language of 'special needs': 'The law says that a child has special educational needs if he or she has: a learning difficulty (i.e. a significantly greater difficulty in learning than the majority of children of the same age)' (DfEE 1997: 12).

This language might be compared with that of alternative definitions which include the historical context and allow disabled people with the learning difficulties label to understand how labelling can be used as a mechanism of social control. For example:

The Government tells schools how quickly a child must learn to do school work and be able to pass tests and what a child should learn. If the school thinks a child is not learning (because of the examination system) as well as other children then she or he will be labelled as having learning difficulties. The problem is that the Government and schools think that learning is based on passing tests. But it is the school who cannot give you school work that you can do. It is the system which makes children learn at one pace. It is the school who cannot find a way of helping you learn. It is not your problem.

(Aspis 1995)

This gives an explanation of why disabled people are segregated within society and continue to struggle for civil rights and deinstitutionalization.

## Choices

Without knowledge of the thinking behind social structures which have damaged so many disabled people, such as institutionalization and eugenics, it is difficult to challenge practice in a meaningful way. However, it is not just the withholding of information but the way in which the information which *is* given is framed, usually in 'positive' language, as 'the facts'. For example, jargon-free literature informs disabled people with the learning difficulties label that services such as day centres and group homes are there to provide 'support'; language like this can act like a magnet, especially for those who feel oppressed.

In the Open University pack (1996: 24), one of the questions asked was 'What makes it possible for people [with learning difficulties] like Pat and Mabel to live in the community? Record your ideas.' Then, in apparent answer to the question it suggests:'Did you think of group homes, foster families, hostels, supported living, training centres, supported employment, families, schools and benefits?', which are all indicative of dependency. This is emphasized by what is missing from the list: community opportunities such as work, education, inclusive politics and leisure, and living in your own home with or without support (thus indicating that there is a choice). These are opportunities which need to be created and supported, as opposed to those which can be given in form of institutionalized 'support' services. There is, further, no information provided on how these opportunities and choices can be created and where to find *appropriate* support in creating them, nor is anything said about refusing opportunities which are offered because they are not appropriate.

## Individual and collective rights

Jargon-free publications frequently contain references to making choices, but there is a point at which simplicity becomes confusion, for example where choices become linked to 'rights'. Consider the following two statements from the same page of Gooding (1991: 12, italics added):

- I *have the rights* to make my own choices.
- We need information that is easy to understand so we can *make the right* choices.

Firstly, there are two phrases – 'the rights' and 'the right choices' – which mean very different things, but which both contain the word 'right'. There is therefore no clear distinction between the rights a person *should* have, which are often moral rights, and *does* have (legal rights), which confuses and distorts *the concept* of rights. This confusion can also be found in People First publications such as *Everything You Ever Wanted to Know about Safe Sex* (1996):

*Sex – Our Rights*
We have the right to:
- Have information about our bodies and how they work.
- Have information on sex and learn about sex.
- Be treated like adults.
- Have sex with whoever we want to if we both agree.
- Have privacy – somewhere to meet, like our bedroom, where nobody will enter.

The listed rights are ideal rather than real rights because current legislation does not permit a disabled woman labelled as having 'severe learning difficulties' to enter into a sexual relationship with a man. Further, no one can enter into a heterosexual relationship until both consenting parties are over the age of 16, and for a gay relationship both men have to be over the age of 18. It is also interesting that there is no mention of, for example, the right *not* to be sexually abused, which *is* a right in law, even if the mechanisms of the legal system frequently fail to protect or defend disabled people with learning difficulties who have been abused because 'they don't know, can't remember, or don't understand what has happened to them'.

Another example can be found in the *Black People First Conference Report* (People First 1993: 12–13), where there is a description of the rights Black people (should) have:

*I Have the Right:*
- To be treated the same as everybody else;
- To have support;
- To speak for myself (in my own language);
- To have a relationship.

Here, there is no mention of the Race Relations Act and the Commission for Racial Equality which can, in theory, help Black people whether they have the learning difficulty label or not to challenge unfair treatment on the grounds of being Black. Without making an explicit attempt to highlight whether the stated rights are morally or legally enforceable, the reader remains ignorant. If it is true that disabled people with the learning difficulties label have all these rights then why are there so many campaigns to get the law changed?

In all the jargon-free literature, the emphasis is on *I* rather than *we*, giving the impression that the onus is on the individual, rather than group advocacy and collective empowerment, for example, to obtain legally enforceable rights and political change. History – through the experience of women, Black people and, now, disabled people – tells us that it is when groups of people identify with each other and collectively define their oppression that they become successful in claiming their rights. The denial of this in the lives of disabled people with the learning difficulties label, through the language of omission and the reinforcement of ignorance, is the cruellest infringement of rights.

## Conclusion

When examining the range of jargon-free literature, I have shown how much important information is omitted from the text in order to reinforce acceptance of the status quo. The inclusion of information about why people are labelled, definitions of oppression, the power of statutory and service agencies, and the legislative framework would go a long way towards empowering disabled people with the learning difficulties label. The omission of such information is not always deliberate, because there are inevitably those who genuinely lack awareness and understanding of the issues, or who really believe that they will overload, or even hurt us with too much information. Usually our 'support' comes from people from a public service or therapeutic background where the emphasis is on rehabilitation and community care programmes for individual people, and these are the very people who have often not had the opportunity to examine the amount of power they have in this 'support' role because it is disguised with language that is intended to make us feel good and positive – the language of caring and kindness. But where people who possess knowledge and political understanding of the oppression of particular groups of people lack the will to explain this to disabled people with the learning difficulties label, it simply becomes an extension of our oppression.

At the root of this problem are very often low expectations of what disabled people with the learning difficulties label can understand, together with a particular liking for the short-cuts that language enables. These things perpetuate the myth of the 'unquestionable' value of simple language and encourage ignorance of the limits to life experience imposed by the practices of institutionalization and other kinds of social exclusion. Disabled people with the learning difficulties label are not encouraged to understand the subtleties of personal and political relationships and language within compulsory education. Consequently, concepts as well as words are simplified. This compounds the difficulty of providing real jargon-free information which is relevant to our experiences and promotes our empowerment. However, like everyone else, many disabled people with the learning difficulties label have the ability to learn and understand the nature of their relationships and rights if they are supported in doing so. It remains the case that it is not in the interests of many of those who claim to support us to provide this particular kind of support, because it would change the power balance in the relationship between us and them which would mean different structures and ways of working which bear no resemblance to those to which they are accustomed. The responsibility therefore lies largely on the shoulders of the disability movement to close the gap of omission and silence.

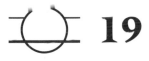 **19**

# Final accounts and the parasite people

## Mike Oliver

### Introduction

The dominant discourse of social research for as long as it has been recognized as an appropriate means of knowledge production has been that of 'research as investigation'. This discourse has sustained my own research over the last 25 years, but as I became increasingly uncomfortable with my own role as a social researcher, I became correspondingly uncertain about the discourse of research as investigation. Accordingly, in critically exploring both the history and development of research on disability (Oliver 1992) and my own experience of it and within it (Oliver 1997), I have come to the conclusion that if we are to eventually develop a truly emancipatory research paradigm, we must ensure that the discourse on which it is based is also emancipatory. For me that involves creating a new discourse which is based upon the idea of research as production. It is these final steps in my own intellectual journey that I attempt to trace in this chapter.

### Setting the scene

The title is not deliberately provocative: it attempts to pay some of my debts to the history of disability research as well as express my future intentions in respect of it. The term 'parasite' is used advisedly and harks back to a pioneering paper by Paul Hunt, who criticized two action researchers, Eric Miller and Geraldine Gwynne, because they failed to engage with the action in producing a research report on the lives of incarcerated disabled people. 'Final accounts' refers to my personal decision not to undertake any further disability research and hence is my final public statement on the issue of emancipatory research.

The *Shorter Oxford Dictionary* defines 'parasite' in two ways: 'animal or plant living in or on another', and 'self-seeking hanger on'. Any of you who have read Hunt's paper (1981) will be in no doubt which meaning of the term he was using when discussing the work of Miller and Gwynne (1975). He was understandably vitriolic in his condemnation of their detachment and objectivity and their failure to side with the residents of Le Court Cheshire home in their struggle against an oppressive regime under which they were living; he was understandably vitriolic because people's lives were at stake.

The problem with his critique, or rather subsequent interpretations of his critique including my own (Oliver 1992) and others (Stone and Priestley 1996), is that we assumed that the solution to parasitic research was commitment: namely that researchers had to give up the pursuit of objectivity in researching oppression and decide whose side we were on. This solution confused, or rather, only dealt with one of the two different meanings of the term 'objectivity': the first seeing objectivity as value freedom and detachment from research subjects; the second seeing oppression as being 'objectively' structured by the social and material relations of capitalism. While I'm not denying the importance of commitment, we have ignored and continue to ignore the objective structures of oppression in much disability research. In my view oppression does not merely exist in the thoughts and actions of individuals or groups, but is the product of those social and material relations already mentioned. Therefore committed (i.e. non-objective) disability research must engage with the objective structures of oppression as well as confronting and combatting the thoughts and actions of individuals and groups.

In order to attempt to engage with these objective structures, in this chapter I shall be defining 'parasite' accordingly, as 'an animal living on another'. To put it objectively (or at least non-pejoratively), disability researchers are parasitic upon disabled people, for without the host body (disabled people) there would be no disability researchers. This is not a thinly veiled personal attack but an attempt to describe accurately the social and material relations of research production.

While Hunt intended to settle personal accounts in his paper, this is not my intention, at least not by naming names. As well as seeking to change the discourse upon which research is conducted, my intention is to challenge the rationale within which most disability research is carried out. To put it crudely, this is how the rationale usually goes: 'As long as I am attempting to improve the lives of disabled people, it doesn't really matter if my own conditions improve at a much greater rate, because my responsibility is to myself, my ethics as a researcher, my funding body or even my commitment to challenging oppression.' These positions are, in the final analysis, never enough, or at least they are not for me, which is why they are my final accounts; I no longer wish to operate within a research discourse which prioritizes investigation over emancipation. The reasons for this will be fully explained as the chapter proceeds.

## The experience of researching and being researched

My own experience both as a subject and researcher (if such a distinction has any validity at all) has led me to some personal pain and general disillusionment with the emancipatory potential of even the most committed research and researchers. This is explored in my chapter in the proceedings of the recent Leeds conference on disability research (Barnes and Mercer 1997). In that paper, I concluded that disability researchers position themselves ideologically in particular ways in order to cope with the contradictions of working between the social and material relations of research production. However, since writing it I have come to realize that I cannot leave matters where I left them – between a rock and a hard place, so to speak. Final accounts always have to be settled, although not in a personally antagonistic way by naming names and ridiculing individual ideological positioning. In this chapter I intend to close my own research account, although I may also suggest ways in which others may seek to open new accounts based upon the discourse of research as production.

In closing my own account it is important that I acknowledge that I am not the only researcher to experience pain and disillusionment about our research, but others have usually been able to resolve their discontent in one of two ways; one I shall call the experiential and the other the participatory approach. I shall deal with both in some detail shortly but here I wish to state that personally I have trouble with both of these attempts at resolution.

Firstly, I have worked within both approaches myself: to put it colloquially, I've been there, seen the video and got the teeshirt. In being critically reflexive about this work, I am led to the conclusion, which I have already stated many times (Oliver 1992, 1996a, 1997), that I am the main beneficiary of this work. I'm not being falsely modest about my contribution to the production of knowledge about disability, the lives of disabled people and even the progress of humanity, nor am I being 'naive or disingenuous' as has been claimed (Shakespeare 1997: 187) because I have never said that I am the sole beneficiary of my own work. Nevertheless, my own work leaves me confronted with a certain amount of existential guilt which I cannot ignore or wish away.

Secondly, these approaches don't confront the objective structures of oppression. As an undergraduate I was taught about what was called the Miliband–Poulantzas debate, which in my view is not merely an argument between British and French intellectuals, but goes to the heart of current debates about power and oppression. For those not as old as I or with no background in sociology, what was at issue was whether power resides in individuals and groups or whether it resides in social structures, and consequently whether oppression is something people willingly choose to do to each other or whether social structures can be oppressive in themselves.

It's no longer fashionable to believe in oppressive structures both because of the current state of social theory and because of the problems of 'what to do' for those who do believe in structures. The decline of Marxism and the rise of postmodernism has enabled researchers to solve their theoretical and individual difficulties at a stroke; postmodern theory eschews structures and allows researchers to continue to produce their own stilted forms of knowledge without cognitive dissonance. Poulantzas may have killed him-self, and for me existential guilt remains, but investigatory social research continues and yet more experience is colonized.

## Experiential accounts

The first of these approaches prioritizes and privileges individual experience above ethics, methodology, objectivity and even sometimes the funding body. While I have considerable sympathy with this approach, one problem is that it often assumes that providing faithful accounts of individual experience is enough. Of course it never is, as many Chicago interactionists, medical soci-ologists and standpoint feminists could testify if they had been reflexively critical of their own work. Another problem is a methodological one: the researching of collective as opposed to individual experience. Most of the research techniques involve one researcher and one research subject inter-acting with each other, the nature of the interaction being shaped by the research paradigm within which the researcher is operating. Even ethno-graphic approaches to collective phenomena like cultures or subcultures are still dependent upon one-to-one interactions with key informants. After nearly 200 years of social research we still do not have the faintest idea of how to produce collective accounts of collective experience. A third problem is that the approach can be an exclusionary one, which results in noses being bitten off spited faces because it focuses on a false problem; who is entitled to research experience? This debate about who can and should research experi-ence is usually conducted as if it is the first time the issue has ever been raised, and with such high emotions that friends as well as enemies often end up being excluded.

Recently while reading an autobiography of Woody Guthrie I came across similar arguments to those currently raging in disability research, and these were taking place more than 50 years ago:

> When he was most frustrated . . . Woody had a tendency to go overboard and claim that you actually had to experience something before you could write a song about it. He would, in passing, slash sweet, virginal Bess Lomax for trying to sing the whorehouse song, 'The House of the Rising Sun'.
>
> (Klein 1981: 208)

However Woody was often goosed by his own gander in the form of Gordon Friesen, who had grown up on a dirt farm in Oklahoma and was 'authentic-ally' a worker:

> Whenever Woody started flaunting his 'authenticity' and going on about migrants, Gordon would let him have it 'Woody, what on earth are you talking about? You never harvested a grape in your life. You're an intel-lectual, a poet – all this singin' about jackhammers, if you ever got within

five feet of a jackhammer it would knock you on your ass. You scrawny little bastard, you're shitting the public: You never did a day's work in your life'.

(Klein 1981: 213)

This raises the uncomfortable question of whether disability researchers are 'shitting' disabled people when they write about experiences that they have no access to save through their own research techniques. The answer, in my view, is not tied to whether researchers have an impairment or not, but where we position ourselves between the social and material relations of research production (Oliver 1997).

The final problem is that this approach often fails to tie itself to emancipatory theory or praxis, assuming standpoint epistemology is all that is necessary. As Denzin (1997: 54) puts it, 'A politics of action or praxis, however, is seldom offered.' But how could it be in a research paradigm dominated by an investigatory discourse? The researcher's responsibility stops with the provision of an accurate account of experience – what to do with this account is always someone else's problem.

## Participatory accounts

The second approach calls for participatory strategies involving research subjects. It attempts to deal with the problem of emancipation by sharing or attempting to share responsibility and indeed blame with the research participants. The worst exemplar of this is the attempt to do participation by employing a few disabled people as researchers, often without much support or understanding of what that means. Next worst comes involving disability organizations (often non-representative ones) in the process of research production. Least worst involves commitment to involving organizations of disabled people at all stages in the research process, short of overall control over resources and agendas.

The problem with all of these is that they do not confront the objective structures of oppression, and despite personal intentions in many cases, disabled people are still positioned in oppressive ways. Whether we like it or not, failing to give disabled people (through their own representative organizations) complete control over research resources and agendas inevitably positions disabled people as inferior to those who are in control. To preview what I am coming on to say, we designate disabled people as inferior by our actions, regardless of our intentions.

When we set up research programmes, persuade our organizations to take a specific interest in disability issues and bid into funded initiatives (and I have done all these things myself) we are instrumental in the production of a particular set of social relations. In settling my final accounts with myself, I can no longer pretend that adopting any of the above strategies is the best we can do in current circumstances or that it is better than doing nothing.

Because of the oppressive structures in which we are located, such actions inevitably keep that oppression in place.

## The need for new accounts

A new epistemology for research praxis is necessary, and it must be one which goes beyond standpoint and action approaches. For me this epistemology must reject the discourse that sustains investigatory research and replace it with a discourse that suggests that research produces the world. This is not new, of course; Marx argued that the class that owned the means of material production was also responsible for 'mental production', and Gramsci suggested that under certain conditions, ideas themselves could be material forces. And finally Foucault refused to separate knowledge from power, arguing that the structures that maintain one also sustain the other.

Research, however, has never really integrated this into itself, and has lived within a discourse that suggests that there is a world out there to be investigated; even Marx himself was reportedly designing a questionnaire shortly before his death. It is very difficult to undertake research based upon the discourse of production, not simply for operational or careerist reasons but also because of the intellectual backlash it is likely to provoke.

At a seminar in Leeds in 1996 Tim Booth was faced by anger and outrage when he suggested that many of his research subjects (people with learning difficulties) were unable to produce coherent accounts of themselves, so it was the researcher's responsibility to do it with them, though not for them. My own reaction to this suggestion was one of anger too, but at that time I had not fully resolved my own reflexive problems with my own research. I had not fully understood that emancipatory research can only be an act of collective production.

Research, no matter how radical, committed or emancipatory, has continued to be based upon the investigatory discourse – my recently completed research (Campbell and Oliver 1996) was based upon my own assumption that I was investigating the disability movement. It is only now that I recognize that I wasn't, even if unconsciously I already knew that. (It's also interesting to note the coincidence of becoming aware of my unconscious in respect of my research at the same time as I have come to acknowledge, for the first time, the role of my unconscious in all other aspects of my life, but that's another story.) To return to my own research, however, and to put it clearly and unequivocally, when Jane Campbell and I researched the collective political experience of disabled people, we were engaged in an act of production, not investigation, even if we did not know it at the time. We were producing ourselves collectively as a coherent, strong and articulate political movement, and individually as proud and committed political actors.

Here I have problems with the terms 'I' and 'we', largely because I have not discussed this with Jane and therefore do not know how much of it is an act of individual and how much an act of joint production. But it goes further than mere personal accountability: just as I pointed out earlier we do not have the methodological techniques to undertake collective research, nor do we have the language to produce ourselves collectively. Thus in the creation of a discourse which sees research as an act of production we will need to develop a new language which enables us to talk about it.

## Research and the discourse of production

This idea of research and indeed other social acts as production has enabled me to think through the challenge Paul Abberley recently presented us with, when he raised the question of what life will be like in a Utopia based upon production and labour for those whose impairments make the act of labour difficult. The answer is both simple and complex at the same time: we all labour to produce ourselves. However, it is not as easy as this because, as Abberley (1996: 61) notes, 'Classical social theories give participation in production a critical importance in social integration; in their Utopias work is a need, a source of identity.' He goes on to point out that feminism attempts to resolve the problem of those perceived as unable to work by redefining 'work so as to include non-disabled women amongst the ranks of potentially non-alienated workers'.

Unfortunately, in so doing, disabled people remain oppressed, as Jenny Morris has consistently pointed out (1992). The solution to this, in my view, is not to redefine work on the basis of including yet one more sectional interest regardless of the consequence to other groups, but to broaden our idea of the nature of production itself. In other words, to return to Marx and the idea that the act of labour does not merely involve the production of the social and material forms of life, but the production of ourselves as well. As researchers, then, we labour to produce ourselves and our worlds. We do not investigate something out there, we do not merely deconstruct and reconstruct discourses about our world. Research as production requires us to engage with the world, not distance ourselves from it, for ultimately we are responsible for the product of our labours and as such we must struggle to produce a world in which we can all live as truly human beings.

There are negative implications to this as well. Do we need to reject the real progress we have made so far in investigating the lives of disabled people? What about the money that is available or may become available to continue to do so? What about the aspirations of disability researchers as well as disabled people because careers in research cannot currently be made out of producing the world, only out of investigating it?

The problem, as I have argued in this chapter, is that our acts of investigation, by their very nature and whether we like it or not, produce the world in a particular way. We can only cease to produce the oppressive world by stopping doing what we have been doing. As Don Juan might have told Castenada, 'It is only by stopping the world that we can truly see.' Once we have stopped the world, the question of whether we have the energy and commitment to do something else instead, to produce a different world, remains.

## Research and the issue of reproduction

In responding to an earlier version of this chapter Paul Abberley (1997, personal communication) suggested that emancipatory research based on the discourse of production might also want to consider the ways in which oppressive structures are reproduced. In so doing he suggests that researchers can avoid 'parasiting the experience of disabled people by focusing on the actions of oppressors'. This adds an important dimension to disability research, and while it is unable to avoid the separation of researcher and disabled people because of the 'objective class privilege of the disability researcher' it nonetheless produces useful knowledge for disabled people in their struggles against oppression.

The emerging sociology of disability has begun to produce just such useful knowledge, but like other sociologies it has also come under the influence of postmodernism. In a previous paper I traced the emergence of the sociology of disability in both the United States and Britain (Oliver 1996b), making the point that mainstream sociology has not taken disability seriously as a category for sociological attention. In this respect, the point that Lemert has recently made about other forms of oppression is apt:

> It has long been recognised that professional sociologists have resisted a serious taking into account of feminism. If anything, their record has been even more dismal in their unwillingness to read with definitive seriousness the writings of other extramural sociologists – the new developments in queer theory and post colonial studies, the varied and serious work by African Americanists, the very considerable literature by and about Black feminists and other women of color.
>
> (Lemert 1995: 207–8)

It is perhaps ironic, even sad and certainly symptomatic of the crisis that sociology finds itself in, that despite recognizing for years the problematic nature of all knowledge, it has increasingly engaged in the production of its own sociological knowledge in ways that have excluded rather than included other interests, communities or individuals, as Lemert (1995) suggests.

It is not merely the use of arcane and jargon-ridden language which has prompted this sociological drift to irrelevance. Nor is it just its failure to move beyond the investigatory discourse of its own research activity. Equally importantly, it is sociology's failure to engage with important issues and debates that are of real relevance to people's lives, coupled with its attempts to distance itself from any knowledge production processes which take the shaping of the future seriously. The pessimistic, postmodernist approach to life as 'survival amongst the ruins' (Baudrillard 1984) appears to have penetrated much of sociology today.

If sociology is to survive amongst the ruins, its survival will depend upon its ability to produce useful knowledge in the real world, whether indeed this be knowledge to assist in wealth creation or knowledge to combat oppression. Engaging in just such a reconstructive project involves not just the reconstituting of sociological theory but a re-engagement with the real world through the practicalities of undertaking sociological research. This will involve developing research strategies which aim to confront the existing structures of oppression by developing what, here and elsewhere, I have called an emancipatory research paradigm.

## Conclusion

Increasingly as oppressed groups such as disabled people continue the political process of collectively empowering themselves, research practice based upon the investigatory discourse and utilizing 'tourist' approaches by 'tarmac' professors and researchers will find it increasingly difficult to find sites and experiences ripe for colonization. Disabled people and other oppressed groups will no longer be prepared to tolerate exploitative investigatory research based upon exclusionary social relations of research production.

Indeed, one could go further and suggest that the production of all knowledge needs itself to become increasingly a socially distributed process by taking much more seriously the experiential knowledge that oppressed groups produce about themselves, and research based upon the discourse of production will have an increasingly important role to play in this. And who knows? This may eventually lead to the fusion of knowledge and research production into a single coherent activity in which we produce ourselves and our worlds in ways which will make us all truly human.

## Acknowledgement

An earlier version of this chapter was presented at the International Conference 'Doing Disability Research' organized by Colin Barnes and Geof Mercer of The Disability Research Unit, University of Leeds, in September 1997.

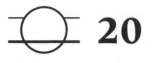 **20**

New disability discourse,
the principle of optimization and
social change

**Mairian Corker**

> If our own political beliefs and commitments are to be seen not
> as absolute Truth, but as insurgent critical discourses, bearing
> the indelible traces of their particular historical and cultural
> origins, then we may be more open to communication with
> significant political others, including the excluded Other.
>
> (Leonard 1997: 143)

**Introduction**

There can be no doubt that disabled people worldwide have been engaged in
a collective re-authoring of our lives which has generated – to poach a somewhat contemporary metaphor – a 'new disability discourse'. One of the critical questions which is commonly levelled at discursive approaches to
understanding this re-authoring is whether they can, in themselves or even
by extension, effectively tackle disability oppression and disabling practices
embedded in the social and economic structures. In this concluding chapter,
I will return to some of the issues raised throughout the book, in particular
those which centre around the production and circulation of meaning
within the field of disability studies, which provide us with some answers. In
doing this, I do not intend to use an analytical approach that perpetuates the
problems which can be experienced in putting together an international
volume such as this one. As examples, we might take the difficulties of
marrying up terms such as 'critical discourse analysis' and 'rhetoric', both of
which have been used in the preceding pages with some overlap of meaning
and some cultural dissonance and/or entrenchment; or the terms 'disabled
people' and 'learning disability' and 'people with disabilities' and 'mental
retardation', which are used differently within and without the disabled
people's movement (disability rights movement, or disability movement).
The issue of linguistic and cultural differences is clearly a significant one

which disabled people are already addressing, but it goes well beyond the 'nice' words and the 'nasty' words relating to disability that are in cultural circulation. Indeed, to view language only in these terms is to take a monologic view of discourse, when even within monologues meaning is contextualized in different ways which interact with each other. Even if we were to find consistent language which was acceptable to all disabled people, we would still not fully account for the different ways that language operates within discursive practice, and it is here that language is critically linked to issues of knowledge, and ultimately power, because particular forms of knowledge are privileged.

Historical evidence relating to minority languages and language varieties suggests that for new disability discourse to produce the kind of sociocultural change which is its task, it must significantly increase both its *prestige* and its *status* by directly engaging with hegemonic structures and practices. Aspis hints at this in Chapter 18. Direct engagement will involve the 'reinstitutionalization and relegitimation of its domain context' – particularly in those cultural domains which are critical for direct social reproduction, such as work, administration and so on – which in turn will have implications for its *corpus* or linguistic features (G. Williams 1992: 147). There are two main ways in which we can conceptualize this process in relation to new disability discourse. First, we can envisage a situation where new disability discourse replaces the state language of disability oppression as a consequence of political change. In this case we need to turn our attention to matters of standardization, specifically *whose* standards are adopted, and other features of the corpus in order to assess the political effectiveness of new disability discourse. Second, a Marxist perspective might be that new disability discourse is produced by the social or class structure and can achieve the necessary status only if the capitalist system which is the basis of this structure is eliminated. This can be achieved largely through the increased status of the 'social group' or 'class fraction' – disabled people and their allies – which uses new disability discourse. Social model theory is strategically concentrated on the latter while attempting to influence the kind of political change needed for the former.

However, initially I want to focus this chapter on the first strategy, which is more directly related to discursive practice, by considering the issues of language standardization and corpus both of new disability discourse itself and of the state language of disability oppression. This is because recent studies in the political economy of language (Gal 1989; Bourdieu 1991) have demonstrated that standardization has a crucial role in upholding and enforcing the power structure in a given society. In order to understand how this happens, it is therefore important to reference key terms which are circulating within both new disability discourse and the state language of disability oppression: disability, impairment and chronic illness. To assist this process, much of the analysis in this chapter will draw on two publications: Mike Oliver's essay 'Defining impairment and disability' (Oliver 1996b) and Simi Linton's (1998) 'Reassigning meaning' which is taken from her book *Claiming Disability*. I have

chosen these texts primarily because they represent two recent, but culturally dissimilar explorations of language and meaning from within the disabled people's movement (disability movement, disability rights movement),
and because they are focused on some of the key meanings which are circulating within disability studies. It is also my view that both authors have
sought to engage with discourses of other oppressed groups in a constructive
way, though from somewhat different positions. After critically analysing
these texts, I will then, in the latter part of the chapter, return to the implications of knowledge production and consumption for disability theory and
disability politics.

## Two stories of disability

The purpose of Oliver's article is to examine 'the articulation of conflicting
definitions of chronic illness, impairment and disability' (1996b: 39), and
specifically to examine 'external criticisms [of the social model] from medical sociologists . . . and from disabled people themselves' (p. 40). He argues
that a partial resolution might be achieved 'by focusing on what disabled
people would call impairment and medical sociologists would call chronic illness' (p. 40), implying that the reason for this distinction is related to the disabling effects of language:

> the term chronic illness is for many [disabled] people an unnecessarily
> negative term, and discussions of suffering in many studies have had the
> effect of casting disabled people in the role of victim . . . increasingly the
> disability movement throughout the world is rejecting approaches based
> upon the restoration of normality and insisting on approaches based
> upon the celebration of difference . . . From rejections of the 'cure',
> through critiques of supposedly therapeutic interventions such as con
> ductive education, cochlea implants and the like, and onto attempts to
> build a culture of disability based on pride, the idea of 'normality' is
> increasingly coming under attack.
>
> (pp. 43–4)

However, later in the article he says that 'the social model is not an attempt
to deal with the personal restrictions of impairment [which] properly belong
within either the individual model of disability (which is widely acknowledged as being historically responsible for disabled people's political and
social isolation) or the social model of impairment (which has yet to be conceptualised)'. He sees the social model as 'contributing to' rather than 'substituting for' an 'adequate social theory of disability . . . [which] must contain a
[separate] theory of impairment' (p. 50). His main reasons for a conceptual
separation are that 'collectivising the experiences of impairment is a much
more difficult task than collectivising the experience of disability' (p. 51), and
the continued existence of 'the hegemony of the individual model of disability'. Hence, 'engaging in public criticism [of the social model] may not

broaden and refine the social model; it may instead breathe new life in the individual model with all that means in terms of increasing medical and therapeutic interventions into areas of our lives where they do not belong' (p. 52).

What Oliver traces, then, is a re-authoring of disabilities as culturally defined individual experiences (plural), which within new disability discourse are called impairments, to disability as a collective noun created from a shared experience (singular) of social oppression. This, drawing on the introduction, is achieved in two main ways:

- by splitting off impairment, which is viewed as negative, from disability. This is sometimes achieved through a conflation of impairment with chronic illness, which locates impairment in an uncertain position in relation to both disability and 'normality'. However, more often the tendency is to locate impairment *in opposition to* the discourse of normality – to regard it as Other;
- by the social model's conceptualization of disability as a structural and/or material *process*, which makes the objectification of our oppression possible through much the same processes that allow our oppressors to objectify us and our impairments. In this way, disability has nothing to do with identity.

Of course, not all disabled people will agree with this analysis. Shakespeare, for example, says that 'disability is a very powerful identity, and one which has the potential to transcend other identities' (1996: 109). Further, the chapters which make up the second part of this book illustrate that disability identity is imbued with multiple and fluid meanings which reflect and create context. However, the social model is not about (reductionist) identity politics.

Simi Linton (1998) also notes this progression, but defines it more explicitly in terms of 'the *linguistic conventions* that structure the meanings assigned to disability and the patterns of response to disability that emanate from, or are attendant upon those meanings'. She, in common with Shakespeare (1996) and others, re-authors disability 'as a marker of [a minority] identity [that] has been used to build a coalition of people with significant impairments' (p. 12). The aim is therefore to 'divest disability of its current meaning' (p. 10) by 'placing disability at the centre' and 'reassigning meaning' rather than choosing 'a new name'. However, Linton notes that 'in retaining *disability* we run the risk of preserving the medicalized ideas attendant upon it in most people's idea of disability' (p. 31), whereas Oliver suggests that this risk comes from 'engaging in public criticism of the social model'.

Both Oliver and Linton agree that hegemonic discourses of disability are underpinned by 'the concept of normality and the assumption that disabled people want to achieve this normality' (Oliver 1996b: 44), which leads to a power differential. However, Linton points both to the 'instability and relational nature of the designations *normal* and *abnormal*, [which] are used as absolute categories', and to 'the relationship between abnormality and disability [which] accords to the nondisabled the legitimacy and potency denied to disabled people' (Linton 1998: 24). She also goes further than Oliver in attempting to define this 'relational nature':

> as the notion of *normal* is applied in social science contexts and certainly in general parlance, it implies its obverse – *abnormal* – and they both become value laden . . . Despite the instability and relational nature of the designations *normal* and *abnormal*, they are used as absolute categories. They have achieved their certainty by association with empiricism, and they suffer from empiricism's reductive and simplifying tendencies . . . The relationship between abnormality and disability accords to the nondisabled the legitimacy and potency denied to disabled people.
>
> (pp. 22–4, author's italics)

Thus she echoes Davis's (1995: 49) view that 'the implications of the hegemony of normalcy are profound and extend into the very heart of cultural production'. But she also gets caught up in the paradox this creates. She accepts 'the relational nature of the designations *normal* and *abnormal*' and that 'race and gender are not perfect terms because they retain biological meanings' (Linton 1998: 31). She also points to the usefulness of Rosemarie Garland Thomson's (1997) terms 'the normate' and 'non-disabled' in 'marking the unexamined centre' (Linton 1998: 24). However, in her later assertion that she is 'not willing or interested in erasing the line between disabled and non-disabled [because] *dis*- is the semantic reincarnation of the split between disabled and non-disabled people in society' (p. 31) she implies discrete boundaries between disabled and non-disabled. While this may be more in line with Oliver's views, to my mind it creates semantic confusion around the 'relational nature' of these terms which seems to contradict her earlier argument. This is reinforced, I feel, when Linton moves on to make some rather questionable comparisons, for example, that between 'the normal' and 'the hearing impaired.'

I do not wish to labour the criticism of these confusions and conflations because it illustrates perfectly Linton's own view that 'setting up these dichotomies' (and disabled–non-disabled is such a dichotomy) 'avoids concrete discussion of the ways in which [people] actually differ' (1998: 23), but dismantling them lays us open to the full potential and power of 'linguistic conventions' and their subversion. Moreover she, rightly in my view, identifies that what might help 'is the naming of the political category in which disability belongs', though this might more accurately be phrased as *re-naming*. The social model has achieved 'the naming' of the political category 'disability', but, as Linton and Oliver agree, this 'naming' suffers from its continued association with hegemonic discourse. By corollary, however, precisely because of the different values and privileges assigned by hegemonic discourses, what neither Oliver nor Linton seems to accept is that this applies to any definition – including the axes 'disabled–non-disabled', 'pride–prejudice' and 'disability–impairment' – which rests upon the dichotomizing of experience, since such dichotomies, in their invoking of the pursuit of equality, become neither 'politically efficacious nor ontologically meaningful' (Colebrook 1997: 27) within a framework of social creation. Again, Simone Aspis's chapter springs to mind.

## Using discourse

What is clear from this comparison is that on the one hand we have a *radical modernism* 'which views the sad effects of totalization as a social failure under certain historical conditions, but not as an inherent flaw of modernity itself' and which 'seeks critically to discover the liberating potential of modern culture' in its focus on structures (Lemert 1997: 40). This sees language as a threat because it becomes no longer easy to think in the simple terms of dichotomized experience and clear boundaries once we begin to view language as discursive. On the other hand, Lemert points to an approach which is more reminiscent of *radical postmodernism* , and is particularly illustrated by the perspective, epitomized in Lyotard's *The Postmodern Condition: A Report on Knowledge* (1984), that

> Science and other forms of knowledge depend on the legitimacy in which the culture holds them. Modernity, thus, is that culture which believes certain *metanarratives*, or widely shared stories, about the value and 'truth' of science, and truth itself. This is an important way in which science is discourse. In short, then, postmodernity is that culture in which those metanarratives are no longer considered completely legitimate and, thus, are not universally held to be completely credible.
>
> (Lemert 1997: 39, author's italics)

It is the latter form of postmodernism, also echoed in the work of Baudrillard, which Mike Oliver criticizes in the previous chapter; but there are others, Marxists among them, who still 'draw upon the insights which historical materialism provides as a method of analysis, but see it now as a historically and culturally contingent discourse amongst other discourses' (Leonard 1997: 142). It is unsurprising, then, that *both* stories contain a confusion of *both* approaches – reflecting the uncertainty of the postmodern age. While I accept completely Oliver's view that we should not try to make the social model anything other than a framework for understanding disability, like ethnicity, gender and sexuality, as a socially created phenomenon, I think there has to come a point where, precisely because it is *not* a social theory, we recognize the limits to a focus on structures. Likewise, Linton's approach does place language at the centre, but does so in such a way that its full force in the production, consumption *and performance* of knowledge is not felt. Again, I think Oliver is right, in Chapter 19, to question research as a process of production and to demand that we we ask exactly what is being produced and why. This is the 'macro-political' concern of the disability movement. But Shakespeare is also correct to remind us of feminism's emphasis on the centrality of local knowledges or 'micro-politics' to the processes of interpretation and the challenge to 'Truth' (Chapter 17).

What I am interested in, as a sociolinguist who falls within the *strategic postmodernism* category of social theory, is primarily in attacking totalizing aspects of modernist essentialism. Strategic postmodernism believes

> that modernity is too clear, too subtle in its workings, for any one to be able to criticise it from the point of view of its own ideas. [Therefore] we have no sensible choice but to use modern culture, that is: to subvert the culture, to overcome its denial of differences, its deceptive deployment of power/knowledge, its self-denying ideologies. Strategic postmodernism wages war on totality by working within the modern, as modernity works within us. As modernity deceives us into ignoring painful differences, [strategic postmodernism] seeks to subvert those deceptions by its own tricks.
>
> (Lemert 1997: 53)

And because I see discourse as being central in this subversion, I am concerned with questions of whether cultural and contextual usage of the same terms necessarily indicates that users in these cultures and contexts are attempting to convey the same meaning; whether giving additional dimensions of meaning to reified terms which are in common usage in one culture or context can always produce the necessary impetus for universal social and political change and, by corollary, whether changing the language necessarily implies social and political change. In the latter case, for example, we might consider whether the proposed introduction of the terms 'inclusion' and 'inclusive education' in the British government's Green Paper *Excellence for All Children: Meeting Special Educational Needs* as a general rule implies a change in the underlying practices of locational integration and special education. I am also concerned, as a member of an oppressed minority, with what allegiances are implied (though not always intended) in the production, centralization and valorization of particular forms of meaning, whether these forms of meaning are used consistently, and what outcomes this might have for the task of social and political change. I will come back to this latter point in the next section.

Disability, for both Linton and Oliver, must be placed at the centre of theory and practice or made, in Butler's (1997) terms, its 'proper object'. However, the way in which this is achieved and maintained is quite different from the conceptual splitting of sex/gender, race/ethnicity and sex/sexuality. Though new disability discourse *has* significantly changed the meaning of disability to achieve its discursive and political distinction from impairment, there is, as Linton acknowledges, no distinction *in the 'naming' terminology* used by the state language of disability oppression and new disability discourses. So, in all forms of communication whether spoken, written or signed, disability must be properly contextualized if its meaning is to be unambiguous. However, because a discursively ambiguous term is placed *at the centre* of new disability discourse, this actually makes it very difficult to talk in a nuanced way about disability against a background of hegemonic ideologies. Precisely because disability is socially created, it varies in accordance with the nature of the associated problematic – 'normalcy'. Texts of disability, like any text, are always 'intertextual' (Kristeva 1986; Fairclough 1993) or 'translinguistic' (Bakhtin 1986):

> Bakhtin points to the relative neglect of the communicative functions of language within mainstream linguistics, and more specifically to the neglect of ways in which texts and utterances are shaped in prior texts that they are 'responding' to, and by subsequent texts that they 'antici-pate' . . . Kristeva ( 1986: 39) observes that intertextuality implies 'the insertion of history (society) into a text and of this text into history', by which she means that the text absorbs and is built out of texts from the past [and] responds to, reaccentuates, and reworks past texts, and in so doing helps to make history and contributes to wider processes of change, as well as anticipating and trying to shape subsequent texts.
>
> (Fairclough 1993: 101)

The chapters by Brad Byrom (Chapter 16), Murray Simpson (Chapter 15) and Emma Stone (Chapter 14) incorporate an element of what might be called 'vertical' intertextual relations; that is, there is reference to texts that are 'historically linked in various time-scales and along various parameters, including texts which are more or less contemporary' (Fairclough 1993: 103).

But it is important to remember that intertextuality can also have a 'horizontal' dimension which can be more implicit, as I have tried to show in my deconstruction of Linton's and Oliver's texts. It is here, I would suggest, that the main difficulties arise with the use of the term 'disability'. As an example I would like to spend a few minutes looking at a newspaper article which 'highlights the diverse and often contradictory elements and threads which go to make up a text' (Fairclough 1993: 104). This article (Figure 20.1) was published in *The Independent* on 1 March 1996. This text comprises four main parts:

- the photograph, which occupies 43 per cent of the total area of the article;
- the headline, which is in two parts, one of which is white on black and so stands out more;
- the sub-heading;
- the script.

Though the article is primarily about disability arts, it has a number of elements which together point to the idea of disability being constructed in different ways. It toys with the individual and social models, the relationship both between language and the body and between the author of the text and the subject of the text. From the point of view of analysis, it is important to note that the most obvious textual reference to disability can be found in the *sub-heading* and in the caption to the photograph which highlights deafness *in its association with spoken and written language*, in a positive way – 'Being deaf helps me to explore language as a fluctuating medium.' It only becomes evident through reading the text that the subject's position is to a certain extent contradicted by the author's use of (distorted and negative) auditory imagery.

Now, I want to explain specifically what happened, and has happened since on a number of occasions, when I have used this article in a teaching session with a group of Deaf sign language users. Before introducing the article, I had explained, within a general equalities context, that there were a number of ways of seeing disability, and had included a description of the social model which the group said they had understood. This article was, however, given to the group alongside a number of others which were *not* disability related and offered up as part of a general discussion on inequality. On viewing this article, most of the group, being of 'visual' orientation, homed in on the photograph, which was unsurprising because the rest of the information was in English. The subject of the photograph was variously described by the group as having 'mental health problems', 'epileptic fit', 'a drug problem', 'twisted hands', 'cerebral palsy like my sister', being 'angry', 'unable to control himself', and in more general terms such as 'poor', 'scruffy' and 'untidy'. I then drew their attention to the subtext *Deaf poet and musician*. Their responses were generally of disbelief: 'He's not Deaf', 'He can't be Deaf', 'He's definitely disabled'. I knew what they were saying was that the actor in question was 'Other', 'not-me', because the way that 'Deaf' was signed indicated that they were referring to the cultural meaning of 'Deaf'. Further, because this actor was not known in the local Deaf community, they were also saying: 'We don't know him so he can't be Deaf.' This would also be the case (though not always) if their responses were written, because of the big D/small d convention. I think this in some ways parallels the experiences documented in Susan Gabel's and Judy Singer's chapters, where group resistance is encountered to extended or new uses of 'disability'. However, it is interesting to note that if 'Deaf' and 'deaf' are spoken, it is not possible to tell the difference unless extra explanation is given by way of additional text or emotive overtones, which makes this convention similar to the use of 'disability' in social discourse.

Much of this analysis parallels the recent concerns of Judith Butler in relation to the interface between feminism and queer studies which draws upon Martin's (1994) conceptualization of the problematic relationship between gender and sexuality. Butler argues strongly against certain trends within contemporary theory on the construction of social identities and the tendency to foreground one determinant of the body over others:

> the methodological domain of women's studies is that which 'includes any research that treats gender (whether female or male) as a central category of analysis'. The parenthetical reference to 'female or male' suggests that these terms are interchangeable with the notion of gender, although conventional formulations of the sex/gender distinction associated 'sex' with female or male – or with the problematic of a continuum between them – and 'gender' with the social categories of men and women. This . . . suggestion that gender might be understood as

# Aural anarchy from the sound of silence

## Deaf poet and musician Aaron Williamson gives explosive 'recitals'. **Susan de Muth** was among the shell-shocked

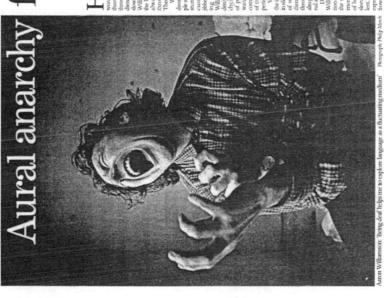

Aaron Williamson: 'Being deaf helps me to explore language as a fluctuating medium'  Photograph: Philip Meech

He stands outside the performance space and peers through the glass doors. He holds up words printed on boards, burns them, throws them at the window, posts them through a gap in weighty silence. The audience strains to read them. The "joke" slowly dawns on those who know: Aaron Williamson has turned the tables on us, the hearing. For he is profoundly deaf, always seeking to decipher words through lip-reading or sign language. There is some uneasy laughter.

When he bursts through the glass doors, it is like an explosion of noise. People slap-back, tread on each others' toes, stumble; we're assailed by the violent cacophony of his roaring, screaming, gibbering, sweeping and moaning. Stamping so the floorboards resound, Williamson strikes a balletic pose and suddenly, from the echoes of his aural anarchy, brings forth a serene and lucid stream of poetry. The feedback from his wayward hearing aid produces an eerie accompaniment which could be the music of the spheres. Some people cry. The experience is overwhelming.

Williamson's subject is his deafness, the intense inner life of a person located in silence, the frustrations and limitations of verbal communication. That the audience participates in this experience through sound and words is ironic, but also part of what makes the work so original and powerful.

Drained by his performance, Williamson happily accepts the suggestion of a few drinks. As we move through the shell-shocked remnants of the audience in the foyer, a girl of five breaks free of her father's hand and tugs at Aaron's sleeve. 'I thought you were really excellent,' she pipes up. A grin, an indulgent expression of surprise sweeps away his frown and he thanks her. 'People don't nor-

mally know what to make of it,' he confides.

The bar is noisy and conversation is harder for me than for Williamson who is an astonishingly adept lip-reader. Although he started losing his hearing at seven years old, he covered it up, staying in mainstream education until he left at 16. 'I heard rejection - social and personal - and preferred not to tell people I was deaf,' he says. He fooled most of his teachers.

At 14, Williamson is doing well. His books of verse, Cathedral Lung and Holophonal Symposium, are sold out and highly regarded. He has a growing following and lectures in Performance Writing at Dartington College in Devon. There is deep rootedness of purpose and self-reliance about him, yet his poetry and performances testify that this was not always so.

Although the adults around him hoped for a miracle cure, Williamson says that he 'knew the truth' at 10. 'I felt the world drifting away from me,' he recalls in a voice that still bears traces of his Derbyshire roots. 'At night I would be secretly traumatised. But I blocked against the initial feelings of terror and isolation. I decided never to accept not trying to communicate as an option.'

With deafness encroaching by stages, cruelty, rejection and "intense hermetic friendships" characterised his teenage years. These eventually spat out a fully fledged punk rocker who fronted a band with his own brand of violently energetic vocals.

Music remains a passion. 'I often wish I could hear new records,' he says, 'but I get a lot out of reading really good reviews.' He still performs with musicians and recently toured eastern Europe with Alex Balanescu of the Balanescu quartet). 'I am keenly sensitive to vibrations,'

Williamson explains. 'I can feel the beat through the floor and I can see the musician's rhythm as they play.'

Pronounced "profoundly deaf" at 27, Williamson changed course. He gave up playing with bands and went to university, where he gained a first-class degree in Literature. He also embarked upon his career as a poet and performer, realising that his unique perspective gave him a lot to say about language in a phonocentric world.

Williamson challenges conventional ideas of what is "beautiful" in poetry. His work explores the inner life not only emotionally, or mentally, but also physically. In Cathedral Lung, for example, he graphically describes the process of forming words - the labour of utterance. 'Tongue/ palls along/ pulleys, tarpaulins and traps ... the whole thing groaning ... a soul slides towards daylight/ funnelling from/ onto the roots/ watches/ hoisting/ the dead mass of dead/ purple weight.'

That this effort is finally futile - the poem ends with the words entering his throat rather than leaving his mouth - is a powerful description of the frustrations of conversation.

The relationship between language and the body is one which fascinates him. For Williamson, writing, as well as performance, should be a radical exploratory exercise. 'English poetry at the moment tends to be defensive of already established positions,' he says. 'Yet there are so many more seams to unearth in language. The words themselves, the modes of saying, are as significant as meaning. I am looking for a more physical currency of accord. My work is restless: "mainstream" nor "experimental". As a deaf person, I haven't made an aesthetic choice, my work relates to actual-ity.'

Although Williamson did not grow

up in the deaf community and does not see himself as a role model or spokesperson, he is intensely aware of social attitudes towards the deaf. 'Even politically correct newspapers say so-and-so was deaf to something,' he says. 'I suppose they mean ignorant. There is a perception that deaf people are bad-tempered, like Beethoven, which surfaces in a woodshow signs of assertiveness or ill-humour.'

The average British male, he says, refuses to facilitate communication. 'I rarely have a problem with anyone else though. If I can't decipher what they're saying, they'll write it down. For some it can be a unique exchange - as if the act of writing were programmed in, so he laughs incredulously. The reticence, he believes, is also class-based. 'The upper classes rely on attracting and controlling people by saying not very much at all,' he notes.

In the past few years, Williamson has developed 'almost constant synaesthesia': sounds from the stock in his memory supersmpose themselves onto visual events - an effect he finds fascinating. Equally interesting are the lapses of communication which occur in personal relationships. 'It's like, oh, there's a misunderstanding, quite a funny one too,' he writes. Intimate friendships however, are treasured and guard him against 'the inherent danger of withdrawal'.

'Being deaf,' he concludes, 'helps me to explore language as an unstable, fluctuating medium. My position as an artist is absolutely my position as a person. This statement is always greeted with incredulity, but I actually prefer being the way I am.'

equivalent to 'female or male' thus appears to rest on a conflation of sex with gender.

(Butler 1997: 4)

What is interesting, however, is that when the linguistic conventions of hegemony are consciously inverted, or the non-realigned meaning of 'disability' is used by disabled people in such a way that it actively reproduces hegemonic discourses, *it can also challenge or contribute to the removal of social barriers*. For example, one of the stories circulating in the disability movement concerns a meeting between disabled activists and government officials where the latter, much to the anger of the former, persisted with the use of the term 'people with disabilities' in spite of having been informed that this term was regarded as offensive. Eventually, one of the disabled activists began systematically to use the term 'people with abilities' to refer to the 'other side'. The atmosphere in the meeting rapidly deteriorated until one 'person with abilities' in exasperation retorted 'Please stop using that term . . . I don't like it!' The response, predictably was 'Now you know how we feel!'

Another strategy is illustrated in Chapter 10 by Mark Priestley, who portrays disabled youth 'as social actors, engaging directly with institutional discourses of disability, and actively reconstituting them to their own advantage'. The language they use is the language of 'normalcy' coupled with a high degree of self-awareness and irony which is lost on the hegemonically acclimatized ears of adults. It could be argued, then, that on a superficial level this is not very different from the 'language crossing' which occurs in multi-racial urban youth culture (Rampton 1995), particularly what is described as 'the use of an outgroup language being cross-ethnically "we-coded"' (Rampton 1995: 59). In the light of this, it would be prudent to consider what the outcome of such negotiation would be, both in terms of language and in terms of social identity, if the irony was missing. In other words, what would happen if the message concurred with the 'sick' role as being the individual's responsibility – 'Please can I leave early because it takes me so long to get to the canteen 'cos I can't walk properly?' – or if the language of the social model was applied, as in 'If you don't allow me more time to get to the canteen, the non-disabled children will get all the hot food and that's not fair!' It would also be worth looking at what happens to negotiating strategies when disabled youth are isolated from their disabled peer group, because a lot of the interaction described in Priestley's chapter could be a reflection of collective in-group behaviour, a view which is strengthened by gender differences in the dialogue.

## The principle of optimization

The point about language ambiguity is that it can be employed by those who have more knowledge in the interests of their own power, and that includes our oppressors (see Corker 1998 for some examples). In relation to disability discourse, this happens in part because both new disability discourse and the state language of disability are heavily grounded in *evaluative* terminology. Oliver, for example, says that 'what is at stake . . . is how to *explain* negative social experiences and the inferior conditions under which disabled people live out their lives' (1996b: 41, italics added), but this is not as convincing as it might be because, as we have seen, the 'negative' is silenced through objectification rather than explained. As Linton (1998) suggests, 'disability' is not a perfect term because it retains biological meanings (impairment) which, for many disabled people, are the bodily and metaphysical carriers of negative representation (Barnes 1992; Hevey 1992; Shakespeare 1994). Within this framework of imperfection, disability discourse must be conceptualized by Derrida's notion of *différance*:

> The figure of *différance* describes a particular constitutive relation of negativity in which the subordinate term (the marginalised other or subaltern) is a necessary and internal force of destabilisation existing within the identity of the dominant term . . . The subaltern represents an inherent ambiguity or instability at the centre of any formation of language (or identity) which constantly undermines language's power to define a unified stable identity.
>
> (Grossberg 1996: 90)

*Différance*, the word invented by Derrida to enact morphologically the experience of slippage of meaning, could be regarded as approximating the English term 'deferral', though essentially the term has no exact translation. *Différance* implies that meaning can always be contested on the basis of *différence* (the French word denoting unlikeness or dissimilarity). When new disability discourse is used to resist negativity, and where positive re-evaluations (such as disability pride) are articulated through slogans such as 'Rights not Charity' and 'new' Chinese slogans (Chapter 14) become the language of this resistance (Morris 1991), the entire process of identity formation and social action is conceived in terms of an optimization framework associated with the freedom of the individual, individually or collectively, to manipulate identities in order to achieve maximum esteem and status benefits. The logical conclusion of this process is that the quest for a positive identity through comparison and linked to the mutually constitutive 'figure of *différance*' leads to the *denial* rather than acceptance of negative identities and language practice. For example, aphasia, which was described by Sue Boazman in Chapter 2, produces particular linguistic idiosyncrasies which are at odds with 'standard' English:

> This is a collective of voices often to be not listened to and often not heard and often not to understand. This is a very readable book – filter from complex to be so easily to read. Each chapter invites the reader to the world-word-lives of people with aphasia. Each title of each chapter show the flexible, empathetic, powerful medium of language – reading and out-pick out issues, when the reader ready to dialogues.
>
> (Ireland, in Parr *et al.* 1997: ix)

There is some pressure on people with aphasia not to express themselves in this way, which reinforces a negative identity. The same is true of non-standard forms of both English and sign language in the Deaf community (Corker 1994, 1997).

However, we need to think of the consequences of this silencing for the understanding of disability at both local and global levels. As the chapters in the first and second parts of this book illustrate, both the experience of 'pride' and the ability to manipulate identities is itself socially created, and these narratives hint at very different experiences and understandings of the power relations in which they are embedded. Anthony Hogan (Chapter 9) refers to deafened people's need to 'carve a space to act', implying that existing spaces are limited, whereas John Swain and Colin Cameron (Chapter 8), in referring to identity formation as a process of 'coming out', make an implicit reference to identifying with a social group.

This means, for example, that if pride is a collective experience then the experience of pride may depend on social (discursive) access to the collective, which itself will depend on how the collective's in-group evaluates those on the outside. Moreover, there are clearly very significant differences in the knowledge that disabled people have to engage in this manipulation and in their ability to act out social practices which signal their resistance. Simone Aspis's chapter (Chapter 18) emphasizes the drawbacks of using terms, such as 'rights', which have multiple meanings not all of which represent positions from which people can act. This is unsurprising given the devious and subtle ways in which hegemony operates:

> The DLA (Disability Living Allowance) pack rigidly constructs and controls the definitional parameters of what constitutes disability in such a way that those who need to place themselves within that definition are obliged to take personal responsibility in turning a critical gaze upon their own bodies . . . What this amounts to is an astounding display of power/knowledge and of the capacity to proliferate discourse in accordance with Foucault's (1980: 51) dictum: 'the exercise of power creates and causes to emerge new objects of knowledge and accumulates new bodies of information'.
>
> (Shildrick and Price 1996: 102)

While positivity (in the form of disability pride) is expressed through a linguistically ambivalent 'proper object', there are hidden dangers. Firstly this ambiguity can be used *within a framework of reductionist identity politics* to mark boundaries – to emphasize separateness and *différence* – as the previous section showed. At the level of language, this happens because within the framework of modernism

> Linguistic theory is concerned primarily with an ideal speaker-listener, in a completely homogeneous speech-community, who knows its language perfectly and is unaffected by such grammatically irrelevant conditions as memory limitations, distractions, shifts of attention and

Interest, and errors (random or characteristic) in applying his [*sic*] knowledge of the language in actual performance.

(Chomsky 1965: 3)

Given *the assumption* of an entirely homogeneous community of 'speakers', which the disability movement clearly is not, it is easier for 'ideal' speakers to stand in place of or claim to 'represent' the views of the community (Barrett 1997: 182). This is something that the disabled people's movement has sought to avoid, with its emphasis on the 'collective' voice of disabled people, because, in such circumstances, there is always a danger that 'ideal' speech becomes another way of manufacturing consent for particular power structures, including those of the state language of disability. The social stereotypes which create dichotomies between impairment and disability can be reproduced through a theoretical paradigm that assumes externally definable communities based on identity categories which fail to describe accurately a social reality in which, for example, people may have overlapping identities which do not fit into category-based communities.

This itself raises important questions about 'community' which are over and above those explored by Oliver (1996a) in relation to disability. For example, should the disability movement be democratically conceived in terms of a disability 'spirit', 'genius', 'genuine (disability) culture' (Sapir 1949) or 'conscience collective' (Durkheim 1933) which might incorporate both those who are 'out', in Swain and Cameron's terms, those who are in the process of 'coming out', and the range of social realities which is suggested by our diverse impairments? In this context, Butler (1993), writing from within queer studies, has argued that by leaving the determinant of 'community membership' purposely vague through the continuing *democratization* of queer politics, the gay and lesbian community is defined in a more open and approachable way which is better suited to understanding the reality of queerness. Alternatively, reductionist identity politics might produce a concept of a community based on some essential nature ultimately rooted in biology and hingeing on the 'genetic' reproduction of the 'mother' language, but which is defined only in terms of this nature. However, this concept is more difficult to grasp because new disability discourses are highly divergent from the discourses we are socialized into using – most disabled people are not isolated from non-disabled society in the way that, for example, many Deaf people are from hearing society. Our language occurs across 'lines of social differentiation' (Pratt 1987: 60), and as such it might be defined in terms of a 'linguistics of contact'. I wonder if this is what Mike Oliver means when, in Chapter 19, he talks about 'collective production'.

Problematizing the concept of 'community' is important because identity politics is constantly engaged in the marking of boundaries. The risk of fragmentation often outweighs questions of allegiance with particular identities and, therefore, social groups (Corker 1998). For example, while the first group of descriptions of the photograph in Figure 20.1 were clearly indicative of impairment (and this term was not used directly), when there was a suggestion that this person was part of the same social group, the group closed ranks and excluded him with the term 'disabled', which, given the accompanying facial expressions and body language, *referred to impairment*. This reinforced the view that *while the group had been given alternative ways with which to think about disability*, when the group's self-definition was perceived to be under threat from negative connotations, they reverted to 'old' and familiar ways of discursive exclusion. Such an attitude is coded by the linguistic and cultural rules of a particular social group, and is frequently challenged in the process of boundary crossing – the condition of postmodernity. It challenges a modernist view of the disability community, the members of which are joined by their use of the language of the social model, but are socially defined in terms of status as 'insiders' or 'outsiders' of the disability movement in relation to how rigidly they adhere to the 'language standard' it sets. This may be of importance, for example, to parents who tread the fine dividing line between 'being disabled' by the same processes that disable their children, and 'tragedy talk' which, though a reflection of the power of medical discourses of disability, itself creates disability. This was explored in the chapters by Judy Singer (Chapter 7) and Dona Avery (Chapter 12). However, rule setting from within the disabled experience can equally work against disabled people in boundary crossing because this involves changes in language domains. For example Cal Montgomery, a woman with autism, says:

> Language is how I interact with the world. It does mean that for the most part, I take things in. (Of course, I have a real aversion to people, in general, though there are exceptions, so I think part of *my 'textuality'* has to do with the fact that the people can be miles and years away from me while I 'listen' to them.) I can, under a lot of circumstances, chatter. It's pretty meaningless, though it sounds fluent enough, and it's not usually particularly communicative. I'm trying to get better at writing, and to do more of it, but I tend to take in more than I put out, by far. Since, until the Net, meaningful communication has required an editor's consent, I tend to feel as if what I have to say isn't 'good enough'.
>
> What they tell us is that most autistic (including AS) people are 'visual thinkers' – there are some who are 'linguistic thinkers' (such as me). I think that's missing the point. What I suspect is that there are many visual and (possibly) some aural thinkers; I'm definitely visual. But at the same time there are many imagistic and some linguistic thinkers. I'm linguistic. As I'm getting older I have to do less conscious translating, but in general, when I was younger, I had to translate everything I saw into words, in order to use it at all, or remember it. As an example, to identify people, particularly under stressful or unfamiliar circumstances, I have to describe them verbally to myself and then try to match that verbal description to other stored verbal descriptions. It's an awkward way of going about it, and from what I understand, *not the way most people do it*.
>
> At any rate, this means I have a constant self-dialogue going on. I suppose this makes it easier to maintain a sense of self. In my early twenties,

when I was institutionalized *because my 'way' was socially unacceptable*, they had me on drugs which pretty much robbed me of all contact, all language ability at some times – I didn't have any sense of myself for about four and a half years ...

(Montgomery 1998, via the Internet, italics added)

What Montgomery is referring to is the dilemma of the postmodern condition – the slippage of meaning – and how vulnerable it is within a society where hegemony remains entrenched in modernist values – in this case those which valorize face-to-face contact over all other forms of communication. Her 'textuality' becomes 'socially unacceptable' behaviour in this language domain. This is the kind of resistance which is encountered by disability activists where new disability discourses translate into different forms of activism which are labelled as 'disruptive' – that is, they threaten to make the safety of modernism more chaotic. The difference, however, is that because autism resides at the interface between the individual and society, the concept of 'social group' is rather more difficult to grasp except in cyberspace, where different kinds of boundaries operate. Cal Montgomery's story shows how critical the social group or collective is to challenging cultural hegemony, but also that the collective itself must be tolerant of difference if it is not to reproduce this hegemony.

While new disability discourse has 'no need of' disabling language, it does, in some circumstances, actively reproduce the language of the state discourse of disability oppression which 'blames the victim' by implying 'an active agent (impairment) perpetrating an aggressive act on a vulnerable, helpless 'victim'' (Linton 1998: 25). However, as Woodward (1997: 319) points out with reference to black politics, though

there are considerable political gains to be made from being acknowledged to possess an identity defined exclusively . . . by histories of unspeakable suffering, the role of 'the victim', while it has become useful in all sorts of dubious manoeuvrings, [has] its drawbacks as the basis of identity.

Or, as Baldwin (1985: 78) himself says,

The victim can have no point of view for precisely so long as he [*sic*] thinks of himself as a victim. The testimony of the victim, corroborates, simply the reality of the chains that bind him – confirms, and, as it were consoles the jailer.

Baldwin, as Woodward (1997: 320) notes, 'cautions us against closing the gap between identity and politics and playing down the complexities of their interconnection' – something which I have explored in relation to the Deaf community (Corker 1998). But this also returns us to Oliver's (1996b: 52) point about 'inadequacies' of social model theory being related to 'how we use it'. Because 'use' is underpinned by discursive strategies, how do we reconcile Baldwin's comments, with the 'use' of the social model? And how do we account for the friction between Linton's view (1998: 22) – that disabled people's narratives of 'coming out' should be told because they provide evidence of 'the personal burdens [of shame and fear] that many disabled people have to live with' and 'demonstrate how the personal is indeed political' – and Colin Barnes's more cynical view (1998), that such narratives provide the fuel for 'the true confessions brigade'?

## Towards reflexivity

Much is made of the theoretical divisions between Marxism, feminism and postmodernism which fracture disability theory, but as Oliver notes in the previous chapter, these are the same fractures which threaten to split social theory as a whole. Disability theory, however, owes as much to feminism and postmodernism as it does to Marxism, and though these approaches embrace very different views and emphases in relation to structure and discourse, there are many ways in which they march to the beat of the same drum. As Derrida's notion of *différance* suggests, our understanding of the way in which disability is produced can perhaps be found within the dominant discourse of normalcy, and it is this which should be the focus of our deconstruction. Thus, all are concerned with resisting hegemony and all are concerned with demolishing the supremacy of the 'ideal' citizen who gains power from the production and regulation of social and economic structures of inequality, and legitimation through his – for he is male – reference to professional knowledge.

This resistance clearly has a number of dimensions which are both discursive and structural; the Marxist 'paradigm of production' and preoccupation with structure has been joined by a 'paradigm of communication' which is rooted in discursive strategies (Leonard 1997). This opens up political discourse to issues of language and difference and their relationship to the unequal distribution of social resources (Fuss 1989; Hennessy 1993). But the success of this marriage depends on the development of reflexive knowledge, and it is this that brings the various streams of disability theory, along with theories of feminism, racism and homophobia, closer together.

> Within the critical theory tradition and critical (as opposed to 'scientific') Marxism generally (Gouldner 1980) there resides an element which provides a connection with postmodern critique. I am referring to *the process of self-reflection* [whereby] a class or other social grouping can develop *reflexive knowledge* of the dominant ideologies which constrain them and limit their freedom ... Emancipation on the basis of self-reflection (at individual and collective levels) ... leads to an interest in language – the discourses with which ideology is embedded ... Self-reflection is a political process which enables a social movement to recognise that its ideas, even though expressing resistance, are still reflections of the social order from which they spring.
>
> (Leonard 1997: 142–3, italics added)

This, to me, is the motivation for developing the discursive strand of disability theory which works, *individually and collectively*, alongside the materialist simplicity of the social model and its challenge to the structural world. In other words, those of us who have an interest in discourse are not waging war on the social model. We are encouraging its reflexive use. But more importantly, we are engaged in a different kind of production – the liberation and acceptance of silent 'voices', new knowledges, and therefore a greater range of positions from which disabled people can subvert hegemony and act in the social and political arenas.

But as long as we operate from within monolithic structures or single-issue identity politics which ignore our multiple realities, we remain the subject of their discourses, and ideology allows us to perceive within texts only those discourses with which we are familiar as subjects, or about which we have been made critically aware (Pollitt 1998). This is a plea for the cross-fertilization of discourses of otherness and a linguistics of contact which I believe to be crucial both to the continued growth of disability studies as an academic discipline and for 'the foundations upon which disabled people organise themselves collectively' (Oliver 1996b: 39).

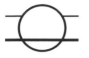

# References

Abberley, P. (1996) Work, Utopia and impairment, in L. Barton (ed.) *Disability and Society: Emerging Issues and Insights*. London: Longman.

Abt., H.H. (1924) *The Care, Cure and Education of the Crippled Child*. Elyria, OH: International Society for Crippled Children.

Adorno, T. (1973) *Negative Dialectics*. New York: Continuum.

Allan, J. (1996) Foucault and Special Educational Needs: a 'box of tools' for analysing children's experiences of mainstreaming, *Disability and Society*, 11(2): 219–33.

Althusser, L. (1971) Ideology and ideological state apparatuses, in L. Althusser (ed.) *Lenin and Philosophy and Other Essays*. London: New Left Books.

American Psychiatric Association Task Force on DSM-IV (1994) *Diagnostic and Statistical Manual of Mental Disorders: DSM-IV*. Washington, DC: American Psychiatric Association.

Aristotle (1982) *The Art of Rhetoric* (trans. J.H. Freese). Cambridge, MA: Harvard University Press.

Aspis, S. (1995) *Learning Difficulties Label Definition Given to Disabled Children in Lewisham LEA*. London: Changing Perspectives in Conjunction with Lewisham Inclusive Education Campaign.

Aspis, S. (1998) *Why Exams and Tests Do not Help Disabled and Non-disabled Children Learn Together in the Same School*. London: Changing Perspectives and Action Research Centre for Inclusive Education – Bolton Institute after Changing Perspectives.

Augustine (1958) *On Christian Doctrine* (trans. D.W. Robertson, Jnr). Indianapolis: Bobbs-Merrill.

Avis, C. (1918) There are no more cripples, *Everybody's Magazine*, 39, August: 62–6.

Bakhtin, M. (1986) *Speech Genres and other Late Essays* (ed. C. Emerson and M. Holquist, trans. V.W. McGee). Austin: University of Texas Press.

Baldwin, J. (1985) *Evidence of Things Not Seen*. New York: Henry Holt and Co.

Barnes, C. (1992) *Disabling Imagery and the Media: An Exploration of the Principles for Media Presentations of Disabled People*. Halifax: BCODP and Ryburn Publishing.

Barnes, C. (1996) Theories of disability and the origins of the oppression of disabled people in western society, in L. Barton (ed.) *Disability and Society: Emerging Issues and Insights*. London: Longman.

Barnes, C. (1998) review of *The Rejected Body* by Susan Wendell, *Disability and Society,* 13(1):145–6.

Barnes, C. and Mercer, G. (eds) (1996) *Exploring the Divide: Illness and Disability.* Leeds: The Disability Press.

Barnes, C. and Mercer, G. (eds) (1997) *Doing Disability Research.* Leeds: The Disability Press.

Barrett, R. (1997) The 'homo-genius' speech community, in A. Livia and K. Hall (eds) *Queerly Phrased: Language, Gender and Sexuality.* New York: Oxford University Press.

Baudrillard, J. (1984) On nihilism, *On The Beach,* 6: 38–9.

Bendelow, G. and Williams, S. (1995) Pain and the mind–body dualism: a sociological approach, *Body and Society,* 1(2): 83–103.

Bentwick, K.K. (1894) Street begging as a fine art, *North American Review,* 158, January: 128.

Berne, F. (1966) *The Games People Play.* Harmondsworth: Penguin Books.

Binet, A. (no date [1916]) *New Methods for the Diagnosis of the Intellectual Level of Subnormals* (trans. Elizabeth S. Kite). Ontario: Christopher D. Green, original French publication in 1905.

Blake, N. (1917) How one man overcame, *The Ladies' Home Journal,* 34, November: 64.

Block, N.J. and Dworkin, G. (eds) (1976) *The IQ Controversy.* New York: Pantheon.

Blume, H. (1997a) Autism and the Internet or It's the wiring, stupid. Paper given at *Technologies of Freedom?*: a national conference on emerging media, May 1997, Massachusetts Institute of Technology.

Blume, H. (1997b) Connections: autistics are communicating, in Cyberspace Cybertimes Section. *New York Times,* 30 June.

Blume, H. (1997c) Temple Grandin: Wiring: an interview by Harvey Blume, *Boston Book Review,* 1 March.

Bogdan, R. (1988) *Freak Show: Presenting Human Oddities for Amusement and Profit.* Chicago: University of Chicago Press.

Bogdan, R. and Biklen, D. (1977) Handicapism, *Social Policy,* March/April: 14–19.

Bogdan, R and Taylor, S. (1994) *The Social Mensing of Mental Retardation: Two Life Stories.* New York: Teachers' College Press.

Booth, W.C. (1994) The five master terms, in R. Young and Y. Liu (eds) *Landmark Essays on Rhetorical Invention in Writing.* Davis, CA: Hermagoras Press.

Bourdieu, P. (1986) The forms of capital, in J. Richardson (ed.) *Handbook of Theory and Research for the Sociology of Education.* New York: Greenwood Press.

Bourdieu, P. (1991) *Language and Symbolic Power* (ed. J.B. Thompson, trans. G. Raymond and M. Adamson). Cambridge, MA: Harvard University Press.

Braithwaite, D.O. (1998) Persons first: explaining communicative choices by persons with disabilities, in E.B. Ray (ed.) *Communication and the Disenfranchised: Social Health Issues and Implications* [forthcoming].

Brannen, J. and O'Brien, M. (1995) Childhood and the sociological gaze: paradigms and paradoxes, *Sociology,* 29(4): 729–37.

Brumfitt, S. (1985) The use of repertory grids with aphasic people, in N. Beail (ed.) *Repertory Grid Techniques and Personal Constructs.* London and Sydney: Croom Helm.

Burgdorf, M.P. and Burgdorf, R. (1980) A history of unequal treatment: the qualifications of handicapped persons as a *suspect class* under the equal protection clause, in W.R.F. Phillips and J. Rosenberg (eds) *Changing Patterns of Law: The Courts and the Handicapped.* New York: Arno Press.

Burke, K.A (1969) *Grammar of Motives.* Berkeley: University of California Press.

Bury, M. (1996) Defining and researching disability: challenges and response, in C. Barnes and G. Mercer (eds) *Exploring the Divide: Illness and Disability*. Leeds: The Disability Press.

Bury, M. (1997) *Health and Illness in a Changing Society*. London: Routledge.

Buscaglia, P.D. (1983) *The Disabled and their Parents: A Counseling Challenge*. New York: Holt, Rinehart, and Winston.

Butler, J. (1993) *Bodies that Matter: On the Discursive Limits of 'Sex'*. New York: Routledge.

Butler, J. (1997) Against proper objects, in E. Weed and N. Schor (eds) *Feminism meets Queer Theory*. Bloomington: Indiana University Press.

Campbell, J. and Oliver, M. (1996) *Disability Politics: Understanding Our Past, Changing Our Future*. London: Routledge.

Chan, W.T. (1963) *A Source Book in Chinese Philosophy*. Oxford: Oxford University Press.

Cheshire, J. and Trudgill, P. (eds) (1998) *The Sociolinguistics Reader, Volume 2: Gender and Discourse*. London: Arnold.

Chiu, M.L. (1980) Insanity in Imperial China: a legal case study, in A. Kleinman and T.Y. Lin (eds) *Normal and Abnormal Behaviour in Chinese Culture*. New York: D. Reidel Publishing.

Chomsky, N. (1965) *Aspects of the Theory of Syntax*. Cambridge, MA: Massachusetts Institute of Technology Press.

Cicero (1988) *De Oratore* (trans. E.W. Sutton). Cambridge, MA: Harvard University Press.

Clarke, H. (1996) unpublished Counselling Diploma Thesis.

Coates, J. (ed.) (1998) *Language and Gender: A Reader*. Oxford: Blackwell.

Colebrook, C. (1997) Feminism and autonomy: the crisis of the self-authoring subject, *Body and Society*, 3(2): 21–41.

Cooey, P. (1994) *Religious Imagination and the Body: A Feminist Analysis*. New York: Oxford University Press.

Corbett, J. (1996) *Badmouthing: The Language of Special Needs*. London: The Falmer Press.

Corker, M. (1994) *Counselling: The Deaf Challenge*. London: Jessica Kingsley.

Corker, M. (1996) *Deaf Transitions: Images and Origins of Deaf Families, Deaf Communities and Deaf Identities*. London: Jessica Kingsley.

Corker, M. (1997) Deaf people and interpreting: the struggle in language, *Deaf Worlds*, 13(3): 13–20.

Corker, M. (1998) *Deaf and Disabled? or Deafness Disabled*. Buckingham: Open University Press.

Corker, M. (1999) Deafness and disability – history, culture and the pursuit of the exotic, in S. Riddell, H. Wilkinson and N. Watson (eds) *Disability and Culture*. London: Longman.

Couser, G.T. (1997) *Recovering Bodies: Illness, Disability, and Life Writing*. Madison: University of Wisconsin Press.

Covino, W.A. (1995) Magic, literacy, and the national enquirer, in W.A. Covino and D.A. Jolliffe (eds) *Rhetoric: Concepts, Definitions, Boundaries*. Needham Heights, MA: Allyn and Bacon, 699–711.

Crawford, M. (1995) *Talking Difference: On Gender and Language*. London: Sage.

Dalton, P. (1994) *Counselling People with Communication Problems*. London: Sage.

Daniell, B. (1994) Composing (as) power, *College Composition and Communication*, 45, May: 238–46.

Darke, P.A. (1998a) review of 'Disability and the City: International Perspectives', *Sociology*, 32(1): 223–4.

Darke, P.A. (1998b) Understanding cinematic representations of disability, in T. Shakespeare (ed.) *The Disability Studies Reader*. London: Cassell.

Davies, B. (1989a) *Frogs and Snails and Feminist Tales: Pre-school Children and Gender*. London: Allen and Unwin.

Davies, B. (1989b) The discursive production of the male/female dualism in school settings, *Oxford Review of Education*, 15: 229–41.

Davis, B H. and Jeutonne, P.B. (1997) *Electronic Discourse: Linguistic Individuals in Cyberspace*. Albany: State University of New York Press.

Davis, K. (1995) A family affair, *Coalition*, June: 5–9.

Davis, L.J. (1995) *Enforcing Normalcy: Disability, Deafness and the Body*. London: Verso.

Davis, L.J. (ed.) (1997) *The Disability Studies Reader*. New York: Routledge.

Dean, M. (1992) A genealogy of the government of poverty, *Economy & Society*, 21(3): 215–51.

Denzin, N. (1997) *Interpretive Ethnography: Ethnographic Practices for the 21st Century*. London: Sage.

Department for Education and Employment [DfEE] (1997) *Excellence For All Children: Meeting Special Educational Needs*. London: HMSO.

Derrida, J. (1978) *Of Grammatology* (trans. by G.C. Spivak). Baltimore, MD: Johns Hopkins University Press.

Deveaux, M. (1994) Feminism and empowerment: a critical reading of Foucault, *Feminist Studies*, 20(2): 223–47.

Devlieger, P. (1995) Why disabled? The cultural understanding of physical disability in an African society, in B. Ingstad and S.R. Whyte (eds) *Disability and Culture*. Berkeley: University of California Press.

Dewey, J. (1926) *Experience and Nature*. Chicago: Open Court Publishing Company.

Dewey, J. (1938a) *Art as Experience*. New York: Berkeley Publishing Group.

Dewey, J. (1938b) *Experience and Education*. New York: Simon and Schuster.

Dikotter, F. (1992) *The Discourse of Race in Modern China*. London: Hurst and Company.

Diprose, R. (1993) Nietzsche and the pathos of distance, in P. Patton (ed.) *Nietzsche, Feminism and Political Thought*. Sydney: Allen and Unwin.

Dirksen, L. and Bauman, H. (1997) Toward a poetics of vision, space, and the body, in L.J. Davis (ed.) *The Disability Studies Reader*. New York: Routledge.

Dowling, M.J. (1917) The passing of the cripple, *Outlook*, 117, 3 October: 166–7.

Dowling, M.J. (1918) A story of rehabilitation by a cripple who is not a cripple, *Annals of the American Academy of Political and Social Science*, 80, November: 43–9.

Dowsett, G.W. (1994) *Sexual Contexts and Homosexually Active Men in Australia*. Commonwealth Department of Human Services and Health, Canberra: Australian Government Publishing Service.

Durkheim, E. (1933) *Division of Labour in Society*. New York: Macmillan.

Equiano, O. (1972) The Interesting Narrative of the Life of Olaudah Equiano, or Gustavus Vassa, the African [1789], in R. Barksdale and K. Kinnamon (eds) *Black Writers of America*. New York: Macmillan, 7–38.

Erting, C. (1994) *Deafness, Communication, and Social Identity: Ethnography in a Preschool for Deaf Children*. Burtonsville, MD: Linstock Press.

Eschholz, P., Roas, A. and Clark, V. (eds) (1982) *Language Awareness*, 3rd edn. New York: St. Martin's Press.

Fairclough, N. (1990) Technologisation of discourse. *Centre for Language in Social Life Research Papers*, 17. University of Lancaster.

Fairclough, N. (1993) *Discourse and Social Change*. Cambridge: Polity.

Fairclough, N. (1995) *Critical Discourse Analysis*. London: Longman.

Fairclough, N. and Wodak, R. (1997) Critical discourse analysis, in T. van Dijk (ed.) *Discourse as Social Interaction*. London: Sage.

Felce, D. (1996) Changing residential services: from institutions to ordinary living, in P. Mittler and V. Sinason (eds) *Changing Policy and Practice for People with Learning Disabilities*. London: Cassell.

Fine, M. and Asch, A. (1988) Disability beyond stigma: social interaction, discrimination and activism, *Journal of Social Issues*, 44: 3–21.

Finkelstein, V. (1980) *Attitudes and Disabled People*. New York: World Rehabilitation Fund.

Finlay, L.S. and Faith, V. (1987) Illiteracy and alienation in American colleges: is Paulo Freire's pedagogy relevant? in I. Shor (ed.) *Freire for the Classroom: A Sourcebook for Liberatory Teaching*. Portsmouth, NH: Boynton/Cook Publishers.

Finnegan, R. (1992) *Oral Traditions and the Verbal Arts: A Guide to Research Practices*. London: Routledge.

Fisher, W. (1972) The narrative paradigm: an elaboration, in B.L.Brock, R.L. Scott and J.W. Chesebro (eds) *Methods of Rhetorical Criticism: A Twentieth-Century Perspective*. Detroit, MI: Wayne State University Press, 234–55.

Fisher, W. (1987) *Human Communication as Narrative*. Columbia: University of South Carolina Press.

Fliegelman, J. (1993) *Declaring Independence: Jefferson, Natural Language and the Culture of Performance*. Stanford, CA: Stanford University Press.

Foss, S. (1996) *Rhetorical Criticism: Exploration and Practice*. Prospect Heights, IL: Waveland.

Foucault, M. (1972) *The Archaeology of Knowledge*. London: Tavistock.

Foucault, M. (1976) *The History of Sexuality*. Harmondsworth: Penguin.

Foucault, M. (1979) *Discipline and Punish: The Birth of the Prison*. Harmondsworth: Penguin.

Foucault, M. (1980) *Power/Knowledge: Selected Interviews and Other Writings (1977–1984)* (ed. Colin Gordon). Brighton: Harvester Press.

Foucault, M. (1988) Technologies of the self, in L.H. Martin, H. Gutman and P.H. Hutton (eds) *Technologies of the Self – A Seminar with Michel Foucault*. London: Tavistock.

Francke, L. (1996) Review of 'Breaking the Waves', *Sight and Sound*, 6(10), October: 36–7.

Frank, A.W. (1997) *The Wounded Storyteller: Body, Illness, and Ethics*. Chicago: University of Chicago Press.

Freire, P. (1970) *Pedagogy of the Oppressed*. New York: Continuum.

Freire, P. (1973) *Education for Critical Consciousness*. New York: Continuum.

Freire, P. (1987) Letter to North-American teachers, in I. Shor (ed.) *Freire for the Classroom: A Sourcebook for Liberatory Teaching*. Portsmouth, NH: Boynton/Cook.

Freire, P. (1993) *Pedagogy of the Oppressed* (trans. Myra Bergman Ramos). New York: Continuum.

French, S. (1993) Disability, impairment or something in between, in J. Swain, V. Finkelstein, S. French and M. Oliver (eds) *Disabling Barriers – Enabling Environments*. London: Sage, in association with The Open University.

French, S. (1994) *On Equal Terms: Working with Disabled People*. Oxford: Butterworth-Heinemann.

French, S. (1997) *Physiotherapy: A Psychosocial Approach*, 2nd edn. Oxford: Butterworth-Heinemann.

Fusfeld, D.R. (1994) *The Age of the Economist*, 7th edn. New York: Harper Collins.

Fuss, D. (1989) *Essentially Speaking: Feminism, Nature and Difference*. New York: Routledge.

Gabel, S. (1993) Intelligence testing: Western ontology and the control of perceived deviance, *Disability Studies Quarterly*, 30–2.

Gabel, S. (1994) Intelligence testing as body ritual, in E. Makas and L. Schlessinger (eds) *Insights and Outlooks: Current Trends in Disability Studies*. Portland ME: Edmund S. Muskie Institute of Public Affairs, 29–36.

Gal, S. (1989) Language and political economy, *Annual Review of Anthropology*, 18: 345–67.

Gartner, A. and Joe, T. (eds) (1986) *Images of the Disabled, Disabling Images*. New York: Praeger Books.

Gernet, M. (1988) *A History of Chinese Civilization* (trans. J. Foster). Cambridge: Cambridge University Press.

Giddens, A. (1991) *Modernity and Self-identity. Self and Society in the Late Modern Age*. Cambridge: Polity Press.

Gliedman, J. and Roth, W. (1980) *The Unexpected Minority: Handicapped Children in America*. New York: Harcourt Brace Jovanovich.

Goffman, E. (1963) *Stigma: Notes on the Management of Spoiled Identity*. Harmondsworth: Penguin.

Goffman, E. (1977) The arrangement between the sexes, *Theory and Society*, 4: 301–36.

Gooding, C. (1991) *Living in the Real World: Families Speak About Downs Syndrome*. London: Newham Parents' Centre Education Bookshop.

Gouldner, A. (1980) *The Two Marxisms*. New York: Basic Books.

Gramsci, A. (1971) *Selections from the Prison Notebooks* (ed. and trans. Q. Hoare and G. Nowell Smith). London: Lawrence and Wishart.

Grandin, T. (1996) *Emergence, Labelled Autistic*. New York: Souvenir Press.

Gray, A. (1921) Joe Sullivan's body is weak, but not his will, *American Magazine*, 91, March.

Gregory, S. (1996) The disabled self, in M. Wetherell (ed.) *Identities, Groups and Social Issues*. London: Sage.

Grossberg, L. (1996) Identity and cultural studies: is that all there is? in S. Hall and P. du Gay (eds) *Questions of Cultural Identity*. London: Sage.

Grossberg, L. (1998) The cultural studies crossroads blues, *European Journal of Cultural Studies*, 1(1): 65–82.

Guisso, R. (1981) Thunder over the lake: the five classics and the perception of woman in early China, in R. Guisso and S. Johannesen (eds) *Women in China: Current Directions in Historical Scholarship*. Lewisten: Edwin Mellen Press.

Gusfield, J. (ed.) (1989). *Kenneth Burke: On Symbols and Society*. Chicago: University of Chicago Press.

Haber, S. (1964) *Efficiency and Uplift: Scientific Management in the Progressive Era, 1890–1920*. Chicago: University of Chicago Press.

Habermas, J. (1984) *Theory of Communicative Action, Volume 1* (trans. T. MacCarthy). London: Heinemann.

Habermas, J. (1987) *The Theory of Communicative Action, Volume 2 Lifeworld and System: A Critique of Functionalist Reason*. Boston, MA: Beacon Press.

Hahn, H. (1988) The politics of physical differences: disability and discrimination, *Journal of Social Issues*, 44: 39–47.

Halliday, M.A.K. (1978) *Language as Social Semiotic*. London: Edward Arnold.

Harré, R. and Parrott, W.G. (eds) (1996) *The Emotions: Social, Cultural and Biological Dimensions*. London: Sage.

Heidegger, M. (1957) *Identity and Difference* (trans. Joan Stambaugh). New York: Harper and Row.

Helander, B. (1995) Disability as incurable illness: health, process, and personhood in Southern Somalia, in B. Ingstad and S.R. White (eds) *Disability and Culture*. Berkeley: University of California Press.

Hennessy, R. (1993) *Materialist Feminism and the Politics of Discourse*. New York: Routledge.

Henriques, J., Holloway, W., Urwin, C., Venn, C. and Walkerdine, V. (1984) *Changing the Subject: Psychology, Social Regulation and Subjectivity*. London: Methuen.

Hevey, D. (1992) *The Creatures that Time Forgot: Photography and Disability Imagery*. London: Routledge.

Hinchman, L.P. and Hinchman, S.K. (eds) (1997) *Memory, Identity, Community: The Idea of Narrative in the Human Sciences*. Albany: State University of New York Press.

Ho, P.T. (1959) *Studies on the Population of China 1368–1953*. Cambridge, MA: Harvard University Press.

Hogan, A. (1995) The governance of deafened adults, *Society for Disability Studies Conference Proceedings*, San Francisco.

Honig, E. (1989) Pride and prejudice: Subei people in contemporary Shanghai, in P. Link, R. Madsen and P.G. Pickowicz (eds) *Unofficial China: Popular Culture and Thought in the People's Republic*. Boulder, CO: Westview Press.

Huang, Y.K. (1964) *A Dictionary of Chinese Idiomatic Phrases*. Hong Kong: Eton Press.

Hughes, W. and Paterson, K. (1997) The social model of disability and the disappearing body: towards a sociology of impairment, *Disability and Society*, 12(3): 325–40.

Hunt, P. (1981) Settling accounts with the parasite people, *Disability Challenge*, 1: 37–50.

Ingraham, C. (1996) The heterosexual imaginary: feminist sociology and theories of gender, in S. Seidman (ed.) *Queer Theory/Sociology*. Cambridge, MA: Blackwell.

Ingstad, B. (1995) Public discourses on rehabilitation: from Norway to Botswana, in B. Ingstad and S.R. White (eds) *Disability and Culture*. Berkeley: University of California Press.

Ireland, C.M. (1990) 'I'm not mad – I'm angry', *Nursing Times*, 86: 20.

Ireland, W. (1877) *On Idiocy and Imbecility*. London: J. and A. Churchill.

Jacobs, H. (1987) Linda Brent: Incidents in the Life of a Slave Girl [1861], in H.L. Gates, Jnr (ed.) *The Classic Slave Narratives*. New York: Mentor/Penguin.

Jagose, A. (1993) Slash and suture: post/colonialism in Borderland/La Frontera: the New Mestiza, in S. Gunew and A. Yeatman (eds) *Feminism and the Politics of Difference*. Sydney: Allen and Unwin.

Jahoda, A., Markova, I. and Cattermole, M. (1988) Stigma and self-concept of people with a mild mental handicap, *Journal of Mental Deficiency Research*, 32(1): 103–15.

James, A. (1993) *Childhood Identities: Self and Social Relationships in the Experience of the Child*. Edinburgh: Edinburgh University Press.

Jenkins, R. (1996) *Social Identity*. London: Routledge.

Jenner, W.J.F. (1994) *The Tyranny of History: The Roots of China's Crisis*. Harmondsworth: Penguin Books.

Johnson, W. (1979) *The T'ang Code: Volume 1, General Principles*, translated from the Chinese with an introduction. Princeton, NJ: Princeton University Press.

Johnson-Eilola, J. (1994) Reading and writing in hypertext: Vertigo and Euphoria, in C. Selfe and S. Hilligoss (eds) *Literacy and Computers: The Complication of Teaching and Learning with Technology*. New York: Modern Language Association.

Johnston, M. (1997) Integrating models of disability: a reply to Shakespeare and Watson, *Disability and Society*, 12(2): 307–10.

Johnstone, B. (1990) *Stories, Community, and Place*. Bloomington: Indiana University Press.

Karlgren, B. (1972) *Grammata Serica Recensa*. Stockholm: Museum of Far Eastern Antiquities.

Katz, J. (1997) Geek backtalk, part II: Geek? Nerd? Huh, *Hot Wired New York*, August: 1.

Kaufman, H. (1918) The only hopeless cripple, *Carry On*, 1(4), October/November: 22.

Keith, L. (1997) His film or mine? *Disability Arts in London (DAIL)*, 123, April: 16–17.

Kimpton-Nye, A. (1997) Shine on! *DAIL*, 122, March: 18–19.

King, A. and Bond, M. (1985) The Confucian paradigm of man: a sociological view, in W. Tseng and D. Wu (eds) *Chinese Culture and Mental Health*. London: Academic Press.

King, Y. (1993) The other body: reflections on difference, disability and identity politics, *Ms.*, March/April: 72–5.

Klein, J. (1981) *Woody Guthrie: A Life*. London: Faber and Faber.

Kleinman, A. (1980) *Patients and Healers in the Context of Culture: An Exploration of the Borderland between Anthropology, Medicine, and Psychiatry*. Berkeley: University of California Press.

Kleinman, A. (1988) *The Illness Narratives: Suffering, Healing, and the Human Condition*. New York: Basic Books.

Kleinman, A., Wang, W.Z., Li, S.C., Cheng, X.M., Dai, X.Y., Li, K.T. and Kleinman, J. (1995) The social course of epilepsy: chronic illness as social experience in interior China, *Social Science and Medicine*, 40(10): 1319–30.

Knowles, M. and Malukjaer, K. (1996) *Language and Control in Children's Literature*. London: Routledge.

Kristeva, J. (1986) Word, dialogue and novel, in T. Moi (ed.) *The Kristeva Reader*. Oxford: Basil Blackwell, 34–61.

Laclau, E. and Mouffe, C. (1990) Post-Marxism without apologies, in E. Laclau (ed.) *New Reflections on the Revolution of our Time*. London: Verso.

Lakoff, G. (1995) Body, brain and communication (interview with I. Broal), in J. Brook and I. Broal (eds) *Resisting the Virtual Life: The Culture and Politics of Information*. San Francisco, CA: City Lights Books.

Lane, H. (1992) *The Mask of Benevolence: Disabling the Deaf Community*. New York: Alfred A. Knopf.

Lane, H. (1995) Constructions of deafness, *Disability and Society*, 10(2): 171–90.

Lane, H., Hoffmeister, R. and Bahan, B. (1997) *A Journey into the DEAF-WORLD*. San Diego, CA: DawnSign Books.

Langellier, K.M. (1989) Personal narrative: perspectives on theory and research, *Text and Performance Quarterly*, 9: 243–76.

Latour, B. (1992) Where are the missing masses? The sociology of a few mundane artifacts, in W. Bijker and J. Law (eds) *Shaping Technology/Building Society: Studies in Sociotechnical Change*. Cambridge, MA: MIT Press.

Lau, D.C. (1979) *Confucius: The Analects* (translated with an introduction). London: Penguin.

Lau, D.C. (1988) *Mencius* (translated with an introduction). London: Penguin.

Lawrence-Lightfoot, S. (1994) *I've Known Rivers: Lives of Loss and Liberation*. New York: Addison-Wesley.

Lemert, C. (1995) *Sociology After the Crisis*. Oxford: Westview Press.

Lemert, C. (1997) *Postmodernism is Not What You Think*. Malden, MA: Blackwell.

Leonard, P. (1997) *Postmodern Welfare*. London: Sage.

Linton, S. (1998) *Claiming Disability: Knowledge and Identity*. New York: New York University Press.

Lip, E. (1984) *Chinese Proverbs and Sayings*. Singapore: Graham Brash.

Longmore, P.K. (1987) Screening stereotypes: images of disabled people in television and motion pictures, in A. Gartner and T. Joe (eds) *Images of the Disabled, Disabling Images*. New York: Praeger.

Low, J. (1996) Negotiating identities, negotiating environments: an interpretation of the experiences of students with disabilities, *Disability and Society*, 11(2): 235–48.

Lupton, D. (1994) *Medicine as Culture: Illness, Disease and the Body in Western Societies*. London: Sage.

Lupton, D. (1995) The embodied computer/user, *Body and Society*, 1(3/4): 97–112.

Lupton, D. and Noble, G. (1997) Just a machine? Dehumanizing strategies in personal computer use, *Body and Society*, 3(2): 83–101.

Lyotard, J.-F. (1984) *The Postmodern Condition: A Report on Knowledge*. Minnesota: Minnesota University Press.

McLeod, J. (1997) *Narrative and Psychotherapy*. London: Sage.

Markel, M. (1996) *Technological Communications: Situations and Strategies*, 4th edn. New York: St. Martin's Press.

Martin, B. (1994) Sexualities without genders and other queer utopias, *Diacritics* [Special issue on 'Critical Crossings', ed. J. Butler and B. Martin], 24(2/3): 104–21.

Mathews, R. (1943) *A Chinese–English Dictionary Compiled for the China Inland Mission*. Shanghai: China Inland Mission and Presbyterian Mission Press.

Mayo, P. (1995) Critical literacy and emancipatory politics: The work of Paulo Freire, *International Journal of Educational Development*, 15(4): 363–79.

Mehan, H., Hertweck, A. and Meihls, J.L. (1986) *Handicapping the Handicapped: Decision-making in Students' Educational Careers*. Stanford, CA: Stanford University Press.

Mercer, J.R. (1973) *Labelling the Mentally Retarded: Clinical and Social System Perspectives on Mental Retardation*. Berkeley: University of California Press.

Merleau-Ponty, M. (1962) *The Phenomenology of Perception* (trans. C. Smith). London: Routledge and Kegan Paul.

Miles, M. (1996) Community, individual or information development? Dilemmas of concept and culture in South Asian disability planning, *Disability and Society*, 11(4): 485–500.

Miliband, R. (1968) *The State in Capitalist Society*. London: Weidenfeld and Nicolson.

Miller, C.R. (1993) Rhetoric and community: the problem of the one and the many, in T. Enos and S.C. Brown (eds) *Defining the New Rhetorics*. Newbury Park, CA: Sage.

Miller, E. and Gwynne, G. (1975) *A Life Apart*. London: Tavistock.

Mills, C.W. (1970) *The Sociological Imagination*. Harmondsworth: Penguin.

Mitchell, D.T. and Snyder, S.L. (1997) *The Body and Physical Difference: Discourses of Disability*. Michigan: The University of Michigan Press.

Mittler, H. (1995) *Families Speak Out: International Perspectives on Families' Experiences of Disability*. Cambridge: Brookline Books.

Moore, H. (1994) *A Passion for Difference*. Cambridge: Polity Press.

Morris, D. (1991) *The Culture of Pain*. Berkeley: University of California Press.

Morris, J. (1991) *Pride against Prejudice*. London: The Women's Press.

Morris, J. (1992) Personal and political: a feminist perspective on researching physical disability, *Disability, Handicap and Society*, 7(2): 157–66.

Morrow, V. and Richards, M. (1996) The ethics of social research with children: an overview, *Children and Society*, 10: 28–40.

Nicolaisen, I. (1995) Persons and nonpersons: disability and personhood among the Punan Bah of Central Borneo, in B. Ingstad and S.R. Whyte (eds) *Disability and Culture*. Berkeley: University of California Press.

Norden, M. (1994) *The Cinema of Isolation: A History of Physical Disability in the Movies.* New Brunswick, NJ: Rutgers University Press.

Norwich, B. (1997) Exploring the perspectives of adolescents with moderate learning difficulties on their special schooling and themselves: stigma and self-perceptions, *European Journal of Special Needs Education*, 12(1): 38–53.

O'Connor, N. and Tizard J. (1956) *The Social Problem of Mental Deficiency*. London: Pergamon.

Oliver, M. (1990) *The Politics of Disablement*. Basingstoke: Macmillan.

Oliver, M. (1992) Changing the social relations of research production, *Disability, Handicap and Society*, 7(2): 101–14.

Oliver, M. (1996a) *Understanding Disability: From Theory to Practice*. Basingstoke: Macmillan.

Oliver, M. (1996b) Defining impairment and disability, in C. Barnes and G. Mercer (eds) *Exploring the Divide: Illness and Disability*. Leeds: The Disability Press.

Oliver, M. (1996c) A sociology of disability or a disablist sociology? in L. Barton (ed.) *Disability and Society: Emerging Issues and Insights*. Harlow: Longman.

Oliver, M. (1997) Emancipatory research: realistic goal or impossible dream? in C. Barnes and G. Mercer (eds) *Doing Disability Research*. Leeds: The Disability Press.

Open University (in association with People First and Mencap) (1996) *Learning Disability: Working as Equal People*, Workbook 3, Equal People: Working Together For Change.

Oshodi, M. (1997) letter, *DAIL*, 124, May: 8.

Padden, C, and Humphries, T. (1988) *Deaf in America: Voices from a Culture*. Cambridge, MA: Harvard University Press.

Parkinson, B. (1995) *Ideas and Realities of Emotion*. London: Routledge.

Parr, S., Byng, S. and Gilpin, S. (1997) *Talking about Aphasia*. Buckingham: Open University Press.

Parsons, T. (1951) *The Social System*. New York: Free Press.

Pêcheux, M. (1982) *Language, Semantics and Ideology*. London: Macmillan.

Pêcheux, M. (1988) Discourse: structure or event? in C. Nelson and L. Grossberg (eds) *Marxism and the Interpretation of Culture*. London: Macmillan.

People First (1993) *Black People First Conference Report*. London: People First.

People First (1996) *Everything You Ever Wanted To Know About Safe Sex*. London: People First.

Perelman, C. and Olbrechts-Tyteca, L. (1969) *The New Rhetoric: A Treatise on Argumentation*. Paris: Notre Dame University Press.

Perez, W., Preston, R. and Andrew, C. (1996) *Not Just Painted On*. London: People First.

Peters, S. (1996) The politics of disability identity, in L. Barton (ed.) *Disability and Society: Emerging Issues and Insights*. London: Longman.

Pfeiffer, D. (1994) Eugenics and disability discrimination, *Disability and Society*, 9(4): 481–99.

Phillips, M.J. (1990) Damaged goods: oral narratives of the experience of disability in American culture, *Sociology of Science and Medicine*, 8: 849–57.

Pinder, R. (1997) A reply to Tom Shakespeare and Nicholas Watson, *Disability and Society*, 12(2): 301–6.

Plato (1984) *Phaedrus* (trans. H.N. Fowler). Cambridge, MA: Harvard University Press.

Plummer, K. (1995) *Telling Sexual Stories: Power, Change and Social Worlds*. London: Routledge.

Plutarch (1983) *Lives of the Ten Orators* (trans. B. Perrin). Cambridge, MA: Harvard University Press.

Pollitt, K. (1998) Deconstructing deafness; public (mis)representations. Unpublished paper presented at Sociolinguistics Symposium 12, Institute of Education, University of London, March.

Potkay, A. (1994) *The Fate of Eloquence in the Age of Hume*. Ithaca, NY: Cornell University Press.

Pound, C. (1993) Attitudes to Disability: power and the therapeutic relationship. Paper presented to The British Aphasiology Conference, Warwick.

Pratt, M.L. (1987) Linguistic Utopias, in N. Fabb, D. Attridge, A. Durant and C. McCabe (eds) *The Linguistics of Writing: Arguments Between Language and Literature*. Manchester: Manchester University Press.

Priestley, M. (1998, in press) Childhood disability and disabled childhoods: agendas for research, *Childhood*, 5(2).

Quintilian (1979) *Institutes of Oratory* (trans. H.E. Butler). Cambridge, MA: Harvard University Press.

Race, D. (1995) Historical development of service provision, in N. Malin (ed) *Services for People with Learning Disabilities*. London: Routledge.

Radley, A. (1994) *Making Sense of Illness: The Social Psychology of Health and Disease*. London: Sage.

Rampton, B. (1995) *Crossing: Language and Ethnicity among Adolescents*. London: Longman.

Randall, W.L. (1995) *The Stories We Are: An Essay on Self-creation*. Toronto: Toronto University Press.

Rheingold, H. (1993) *The Virtual Community: Homesteading on the Electronic Frontier*. Reading, MA: Addison Wesley.

Ricœur, P. (1992) *Oneself as Another*. Chicago: Chicago University Press.

Riggins, S.H. (1997) *The Language and Politics of Exclusion: Others in Discourse*. London: Sage.

Riley, D. (1988) *Am I That Name? Feminism and the Category 'Women' in History*. Basingstoke: Macmillan.

Rinaldi, J. (1996) Rhetoric and healing: revising narratives about disability, *College English*, 58, November: 820–34.

Ringenbach, P.T. (1973) *Tramps and Reformers, 1873–1916*. Westport, CT: Greenwood Press.

Rodgers, D. (1978) *The Work Ethic in Industrial America, 1850–1920*. Chicago: University of Chicago Press.

Rose, N. and Miller, R. (1989) Rethinking the state: governing economic, social and personal life. Unpublished manuscript: University of Lancaster.

Rose, P. (1997) letter, *DAIL*, 125, June: 12.

Rossiter, D. (1990) Personal comment, *Nursing Times*, 86(20).

Rutherford, J. (1990) A place called home: identity and the cultural politics of difference, in J. Rutherford (ed.) *Identity: Community, Culture and Difference*. London: Lawrence and Wishart.

Ryan, J. with Thomas, F. (1987) *The Politics of Mental Handicap*. London: Free Association Books.

Ryan, M. (1990) *Women in Public: Between Banners and Ballots, 1825–1880*, Baltimore, MD: Johns Hopkins University Press.

Sacks, O. (1995) *An Anthropologist on Mars*. New York: Knopf.

Sapir, E. (1949) *Culture, Language and Personality* (ed. D.G. Mandelbaum). Berkeley: University of California Press.

Schak, D. (1988) *The Chinese Beggars' Den*. Pittsburgh: University of Pittsburgh Press.

Scheerenberger, R.C. (1983) *A History of Mental Retardation*. Baltimore, MD: Paul H. Brookes.

Schofield, J. (1982) *Black and White in School*. New York: Praeger.

Seguin, E. (1866) *Idiocy and its Treatment by the Physiological Method*. New York: William Wood.

Seidman, S. (ed.) (1996) *Queer Theory/Sociology*. Cambridge, MA: Blackwell.

Shakespeare, T. (1994) Cultural representation of disabled people: dustbins for disavowal? *Disability and Society*, 9(3): 283–300.

Shakespeare, T. (1996) Disability, identity and difference, in C. Barnes and G. Mercer (eds) *Exploring the Divide: Illness and Disability*. Leeds: The Disability Press.

Shakespeare, T. (1997) Researching disabled sexuality, in C. Barnes and G. Mercer (eds) *Doing Disability Research*. Leeds: The Disability Press.

Shakespeare, T., Gillespie-Sells, K. and Davies, D. (1996) *Untold Desires: The Sexual Politics of Disability*. London: Cassell.

Shakespeare, T. and Watson, N. (1997) Defending the social model, *Disability and Society*, 12(2): 293–300.

Shapiro, J.P. (1993) *No Pity: People with Disabilities Forging a New Civil Rights Movement*. New York: Random House.

Shearer, A. (1981) *Disability: Whose Handicap?* Oxford: Basil Blackwell.

Shildrick, M. (1997) *Leaky Bodies and Boundaries*. London: Routledge.

Shildrick, M. and Price, J. (1996) Breaking the boundaries of the broken body, *Body and Society*, 2(4): 93–113.

Shilling, C. (1993) *The Body and Social Theory*. London: Sage.

Shilling, C. (1997) The body and difference, in K. Woodward (ed.) *Identity and Difference*. London: Sage, in association with The Open University.

Shilling, C. and Mellor, P.A. (1996) Embodiment, structuration theory and modernity: mind/body dualism and the repression of sensuality, *Body and Society*, 2(4): 1–15.

Shor, I. (ed.) (1987) *Freire for the Classroom: A Sourcebook for Liberatory Teaching*. Portsmouth, NH: Boynton/Cook.

Simons, R. (1997) *After the Tears: Parents Talk about Raising a Child with a Disability*. San Diego, CA: Harvest Books-Harcourt Brace.

Skeggs, B. (1995) *Feminist Cultural Theory: Process and Production*. Manchester: Manchester University Press.

Skrtic, T. (1995) *Disability and Democracy: Reconstructing (Special) Education for Postmodernity*. New York: Teachers College Press.

Smith, R.J. (1983) *China's Cultural Heritage: The Ch'ing Dynasty, 1644–1912*. Boulder, CO: Westview Press.

Solenberger, A.W. (1911) *One Thousand Homeless Men*. New York: Charities Publication Committee.

Solenberger, E.R. (1914) *Care and Education of Crippled Children in the United States*. New York: Russell Sage Foundation.

Somers, M. (1994) The narrative construction of identity: a relational and network approach, *Theory and Society*, 23: 605–49.

Sontag, S. (1978) *Illness as Metaphor*. New York: Farrar, Straus and Giroux.

Stanley, L. (ed.) (1990) *Feminist Praxis: Research, Theory and Epistemology in Feminist Sociology*. London: Routledge.

Starr, S.L. (1991) Power, technologies and the phenomenology of conventions, on being allergic to onions, in J. Laws (ed.) *A Sociology of Monsters*. London: Routledge.

Stone, E. (1996) A law to protect, a law to prevent: contextualising disability legislation in China, *Disability and Society*, 11(4): 469–84.

Stone, E. and Priestley, M. (1996) Parasites, pawns and partners: disability research and the role of non-disabled researchers, *British Journal of Sociology*, 47(4): 699–716.

Sullivan, J.S. (1914) *The Unheard Cry*. Nashville, TN: Smith and Lamar.

Sullivan, J.S. (1918a) A plea to the legislators of Michigan, *Hospital School Journal*, 7(4), November/December: 4.

Sullivan, J.S. (1918b) Cripple is elected congressman, *Hospital School Journal*, 7(4), November/December: 8–9.

Sullivan, J.S. (1919) The crippled child's rights, *Hospital School Journal*, 7(6), May/June: 8.

Sullivan, J.S. (1921a) Big aches in little hearts, *Hospital School Journal*, 9(2), March/April: 3.

Sullivan, J.S. (1921b) The old way and the new way, *Hospital School Journal*, 9(3), May/June: 6.

Sullivan, J.S. (1923a) The cripple in the house, *Hospital School Journal*, 11(1), March/April: 3.

Sullivan, J.S. (1923b) Needs of Michigan's crippled children, *Hospital School Journal*, 11(2), July/August: 11 [reprinted from article in Detroit News].

Sutherland, A. (1996) Black hats and twisted bodies, in A. Pointon (ed.) with C. Davies, *Framed: Interrogating Disability in the Media*. London: British Film Institute.

Tajfel, H. (1981) *Human Groups and Social Categories*. Cambridge: Cambridge University Press.

Talbot, M.E. (1964) *Édouard Seguin: A Study of an Educational Approach to the Treatment of Mentally Defective Children*. New York: Columbia University Press.

Talle, A. (1995) A child is a child: disability and equality among the Kenya Maasai, in B. Ingstad and S.R. Whyte (eds) *Disability and Culture*. Berkeley: University of California Press.

Thomas, C. (1997a) The baby and the bath water: disabled women and motherhood in social context, *Sociology of Health and Illness*, 19(5): 622–43.

Thomas, C. (1997b) Feminism and disability. Paper presented at Disability Studies Seminar, Edinburgh, December.

Thomas, C. (1998) Parents and family: disabled women's stories about their childhood experiences, in C. Robinson and K. Stalker (eds) *Growing up with Disability*. London: Jessica Kingsley (forthcoming).

Thompson, J. (1990) *Ideology and Modern Culture: Critical and Social Theory in the Era of Mass Communication*. Cambridge: Polity Press.

Thomson, R.G. (1997) *Extraordinary Bodies: Figuring Physical Disability in American Culture and Literature*. New York: Columbia University Press.

Thorne, B. (1993) *Gender Play: Girls and Boys in School*. Buckingham: Open University Press.

Trent, J.W. (1995) *Inventing the Feeble Mind: A History of Mental Retardation in the United States*. Berkeley: University of California Press.

Tudor, K. (1996) *Mental Health Promotion: Paradigms and Practice*. London: Routledge.

Turkle, S. (1996) *Life on the Screen: Identity in the Age of the Internet*. London: Weidenfeld and Nicolson.

Turner, M. (1996) Review of *Breaking the Waves*, *Disability Now*, December: 19.

Twitchett, D. (1970) *Financial Administration under the T'ang Dynasty*. Cambridge: Cambridge University Press.

Tyne, A. (1992) Normalisation: from theory to practice, in H. Brown and H. Smith (eds) *Normalisation: A Reader for the Nineties*. London: Routledge.

UPIAS (1976) *Fundamental Principles of Disability*. London: Union of Physically Impaired Against Segregation.

van Dijk, T.A. (1987) *Communicating Racism: Ethnic Prejudice in Thought and Talk*. London: Sage.

van Dijk, T.A. (1997) *Discourse as Structure and Process*. London: Sage.

Vygotsky, L.S. (1934) *Language and Thought*. Cambridge, MA: MIT Press.

Waitzkin, H. (1979) Medicine, superstructure and micropolitics, *Social Science and Medicine*, 13: 601–9.

Waitzkin, H. (1989) A critical theory of medical discourse, *Journal of Health and Social Behaviour*, 30: 220–39.

Wallerstein, N. (1987) Problem-posing education: Freire's method for transformation, in I. Shor (ed.) *Freire for the Classroom: A Sourcebook for Liberatory Teaching*. Portsmouth, NH: Boynton/Cook.

Warren, M. (1988) *Nietzsche and Political Thought*. Cambridge, MA: The MIT Press.

Weeks, J. (1989) *Sex, Politics and Society – the Regulation of Sexuality since 1800*, 2nd edn. London: Longman.

Weir, N. (1990) *Otolaryngology – An Illustrated History*. London University Press: Butterworths.

Wetherell, M. and Potter, J. (1992) *Mapping the Language of Racism*. New York: Harvester Wheatsheaf.

Whittaker, A. (1991) *Supporting Self-Advocacy*. London: The King's Fund.

Whyte, S.R. (1995) Disability between discourse and experience, in B. Ingstad and S.R. Whyte (eds) *Disability and Culture*. Berkeley: University of California Press.

Wiebe, R.H. (1967) *The Search for Order 1877–1920*. New York: Hill and Wang.

Wilding, P. (1992) Social policy on the 1980s, *Social Policy and Administration*, 26(2): 30–7.

Williams, C. (1920) *A Manual of Chinese Metaphor*. Shanghai: Commercial Press.

Williams, D. (1992) *Nobody Nowhere*. London: Doubleday.

Williams, G. (1992) *Sociolinguistics: A Sociological Critique*. London: Routledge.

Williams, G. (1997) The genesis of chronic illness and narrative reconstruction, in L.P. Hinchman and S.K. Hinchman (eds) *Memory, Identity, Community: The Idea of Narrative in the Human Sciences*. Albany: State University of New York Press.

Wilson, G. (1989) *Your Personality and Potential*. Massachusetts: Salem House.

Winefield, R. (1987) *Never the Twain Shall Meet – The Communications Debate*. Washington, DC: Gallaudet University Press.

Wing, L. (1996) The history of ideas on autism: legends, myths and reality. Paper given at the Fifth Congress Autism-Europe .

Woodward, K. (ed.) (1997) *Identity and Difference*. London: Sage in association with The Open University.

Yardley, L. (ed.) (1997) *Material Discourses of Health and Illness*. London: Routledge.

Yong He (1996) *Easy Way to Learn Chinese Idioms*. Beijing: New World Press.

Young, I. (1990) *Justice and the Politics of Difference*. Princeton, NJ: Princeton University Press.

Young, R. and Liu, Y. (1994) *Landmark Essays on Rhetorical Invention in Writing*. Davis, CA: Hermagoras Press.

Zipes, J. (ed.) (1987) *Victorian Fairy Tales: The Revolt of the Fairies and Elves*. London: Methuen.

Zola, I.K. (1993) Self, identity, and the naming question: reflections on the language of disability, *Social Science and Medicine*, 36, February: 167–73.

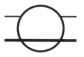

# Index